ERNIE BODAI, M.D., F.A.
AND JUDIE FERT

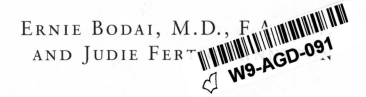

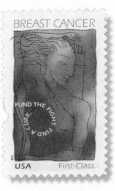

THE BREAST CANCER BOOK OF STRENGTH & COURAGE

Inspiring Stories to See You Through Your Journey

PRIMA PUBLISHING

Published by Prima Publishing, Roseville, California. Member of the
Crown Publishing Group, a division of Random House, Inc., New York.

PRIMA PUBLISHING and colophon are trademarks of Random House,
Inc., registered with the United States Patent and Trademark Office.

All products mentioned in this book are trademarks
of their respective companies.

Portions of "Cancer Compelled Me to Follow My Dreams" from *Thanks
for the Mammogram!* by Laura Jensen Walker, copyright © 2000 by
Laura Jensen Walker. Reprinted by permission of Fleming H. Revell, a
division of Baker Book House Company, Grand Rapids, Michigan.

Library of Congress Cataloging-in-Publication Data
The breast cancer book of strength & courage : inspiring stories to see
you through your journey / Judie Fertig Panneton and Ernie Bodai, eds.
p.   cm.
ISBN 0-7615-6355-5
1. Breast—Cancer—Popular works. 2. Breast—Cancer—Anecdotes.
I. Bodai, Ernie. II. Panneton, Judie Fertig.

RC280.B8 B66568   2002
616.99'449—dc21   2002074302

02 03 04 05 06 AA 10 9 8 7 6 5 4 3 2 1
Printed in the United States of America

First Edition

Visit us online at www.primapublishing.com

CONTENTS

ACKNOWLEDGMENTS

Endless thanks go to the wonderful women, many of whom were strangers, who opened up their hearts and souls to me in connection with the writing of this book. Credit also belongs to the following women who wrote stories on behalf of friends and loved ones, showing that you don't have to have breast cancer to be affected by it: LuAnne McLane, Christina Richter, and Jan Wedge Giuliano.

This book project would never have been undertaken without the insight and support that came from Jennifer Basye Sander, who became an invaluable mentor. Thanks to Libby Larson, the project editor, for her encouragement and attention to detail; to Laura Gabler, for her expert editing; and to Prima for caring enough to publish this book.

I would also like to acknowledge my coauthor, Dr. Ernie Bodai, who is an inspiration to everyone who knows him. He is the perfect example of how one person can make a difference.

And, to the people who make such an incredibly positive difference in my life: my husband, John, and daughters, Leah and Haley. Thanks for your love and support during the many hours I spent writing and learning from these extraordinary and inspirational stories.

JUDIE FERTIG PANNETON

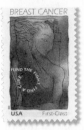

INTRODUCTION

Several years ago I began the campaign for the creation of a breast cancer postage stamp that would raise money for breast cancer research. After countless trips to Washington, a major lobbying effort resulted in congressional legislation authorizing the United States Postal Service to issue the first ever semipostal stamp. As a result, more than 400 million Breast Cancer Research Stamps have been sold since 1998, raising over $30 million for crucial research. The stamp depicts Artemis, the Greek mythological goddess of the hunt, raising her arm to reach for an arrow from the quiver on her back, ready to arm herself for battle. In this case, the battle against breast cancer. Her right breast has been symbolically removed and replaced with the logo: "Fund the Fight—Find a Cure." The position she assumes is that for a breast self-examination and mammography. The rainbow of colors represents the fact that this is a disease that affects women of all colors. In addition, the rainbow is traditionally the symbol of hope—woven into this design, it represents a hope for the cure of breast cancer. The United States Postal Service has championed the cause.

You, too, may now be in a battle—a battle against breast cancer. If ever you have needed strength and courage, now is that time. You, or perhaps someone you love, has just been diagnosed with breast cancer. What now?

You gather up your courage—courage you might not have had to call on before, but it is there. The battle has begun.

As a breast cancer surgeon, I find my job to be extremely rewarding. Each day I meet the challenge of walking a newly diagnosed woman and her loved ones through the battle against breast cancer. Having had cancer myself, it is my hope that my experience makes me more compassionate. I know you are fearful, but I can tell you this: I've had cancer and I am fine.

Breast cancer does not discriminate; it strikes both sexes, all ages, all body types, and people from all walks of life. You will start to see that you are not alone. People around you have been touched by this disease and are available to help you. Don't be afraid to ask.

It is my hope that you can learn from the stories written by these women. Each has courageously stepped forward to offer her experience in dealing with breast cancer. They have done this in the spirit of sharing—so you may find courage. Learn to be strong and learn to be courageous. Learn from Alice Keilson Schnaidt and the inspiring drumming ceremony that her friends held for her before her surgery. Learn from Leslie Mouton, a television anchorwoman who broadcast the news while bald in order to give courage to women who, like her, were undergoing chemotherapy. Learn from highway patrol officer Ramona Prieto, who has dedicated herself to teaching others about breast cancer. Learn from Amy Culp, who decided to tattoo hearts of courage on her reconstructed breast.

Learn from these and many other women that the strength and the courage that you might not feel right now is indeed there—deep within you, ready to emerge, ready to fight. These personal stories will serve as valued friends who have been there before you and are now extending a hand to help you through your own experience.

It is easy to say "Relax and don't worry." But you won't relax, and of course you will worry. Nonetheless, you will get through this. **Be strong. Have courage. Be well.**

ERNIE BODAI, M.D., F.A.C.S.

Bless Me, Lord, and My Bald Head, Too

I've spent the last 14 years in the television broadcasting business. I've anchored in Louisiana, in South Carolina, and all over Texas. I'm now anchoring in San Antonio. In all those years, I've had quite a few hairstyles. Long, short, brown, blond—you name it, I've probably had it at one time or another. But the viewers will likely remember only one style, a style they saw only one night.

The news industry is a competitive one—image driven—and brutal at times. Ratings are what matter most, and feelings are never spared or considered when it comes down to business. Consultants are hired to sift through your wardrobe, analyze your delivery, and advise on your hairstyle. Every time you blink an eye, have a hair out of place, or fumble a word on the air, someone is watching and waiting to correct you. Yet it's not the managers, but rather the viewers who make the toughest critics.

At my current station, every call is written down and every comment noted. Copies are made and distributed. Every day you (and everyone else you work with) see what's being said about you. I've learned that people who like you rarely call, but people who don't like you will call often! It's a business that forces you to develop a thick skin. You can't please everyone, and if you try, the real "you" gets lost in the process.

I knew this particular night would generate a lot of calls. One hour before the 6 P.M. news, I walked into the dressing room and began to get ready. It takes a good 30 to 40 minutes to put on makeup. The harsh lights wash you out, and my skin was already pasty and pale from months of chemotherapy. But the magic of makeup can fool anyone. When I finished, I would look healthy, full of color, and like the Leslie all our viewers are used to seeing. Well, maybe not quite like the Leslie they're used to seeing.

This night, after I carefully glued on the false eyelashes where my own once were, drew eyebrows onto my bare forehead, painted my face with an array of subtle colors, and lined my lips with color, I went one step further. I poured foundation into the palm of my hand and began to rub it all along my bald head. The color had to match my face perfectly. I followed it with powder to keep it from shining under the bright lights in the studio. I looked back over my shoulder and smiled at Betty [my wig]. Tonight, she would stay in the locker. I was going on the air without my wig.

"Five minutes!" I heard a studio operator shout. My heart began to pound.

"This is it," I said out loud. "There's no turning back now." I gave myself one final glance in the mirror.

My friends looked at my head from every angle. "You look beautiful," they said. With that, I walked out of the dressing room and toward the studio. To get there, I first had to walk down a hallway and through the master control room. Person after person gave me thumbs up, patted me on the back, and said, "Go get 'em!"

I stepped into the studio and again was given encouragement by everyone in there. I walked onto the platform where the anchor desk sits, clipped on my microphone, plugged in my earpiece to the control room, and sat down.

"Five, four, three, two, one." The floor director held his hand in front of the camera, the music began to play, and next the open, "This is KSAT 12 News at 6" . . . then the cue. This is where the camera usually has a two shot of me and my coanchor, Steve Spriester. This night it was a one shot of my coanchor. He explained that I would be along in a moment, and then he read the lead story of the day. The second story that night was me. Steve explained that this was a special night, a night when I would share with the public the most private part of my battle against breast cancer. This was the night I would share my story of hair loss. "We want to prepare you," he said. "She will join us for the rest of the newscast, without her wig. It's her tribute to all cancer patients, and a very brave thing to do, too." Steve turned to me, the camera took a two shot, and there I was, for the first time in my life, anchoring a newscast without a strand of hair on my head.

CANCER HAD BECOME a journey of self-discovery that has helped me develop self-confidence and learn to love myself for myself. That was not an easy destination to reach.

It was quite a moment, for many reasons. Mainly, for me, it represented how far I'd come and how much I'd grown! Cancer had become a journey of self-discovery that helped me develop self-confidence and learn to love myself for myself. That was not an easy destination to reach.

When I found out I had breast cancer, I was only 35 years old. I found the lump during a self-exam. It turned out to be a very aggressive form of cancer, infiltrated ductal carcinoma. The good news: It wasn't in my lymph nodes. The bad news: I would still need four rounds of chemo and five weeks of radiation.

The cancer didn't scare me. The surgery didn't scare me. But chemo frightened the hell out of me! I cried when my oncologist told me I would lose my hair. I argued, "No, you don't know. Not everyone loses their hair!" She assured me I would lose it—all of it—and I had to accept it. Why was I so freaked out about the prospect of being bald? As women, we spend so much time and money on our hair. We color it, cut it, style it. If it's a good hair day, we feel good about ourselves. If it's a bad hair day, we feel terrible! (Try a no hair day. I now know any hair day is a good hair day!)

So it was going to fall out. I ran my fingers through my shoulder-length, blond hair and wondered what I would look like without it. I couldn't even imagine it. I went home, pinned my hair up, pulled it back tightly away from my face, and stared in the mirror. I had to come to terms with losing my hair. But I couldn't—not yet. I decided instead of focusing on it falling out, I would buy the best-looking wig I could find and have it ready to go so I wouldn't miss a beat! I went to a wig shop and spent $800 on a gorgeous, real hair, very blond wig. (First time in my life I wouldn't have to worry about roots!)

Then I waited. Two weeks to the day after my first chemo treatment, I stepped in the shower and it happened! Clumps of hair came out in my hands. I stood there, water running down my back, and thought, "This is it." I finished my shower, got ready for work, and glanced into our bedroom. My husband, Tony, was still sound asleep. I quietly walked over to the bed, sat down next to him, and whispered, "It's happened, Tony. Today's the day. My hair has started falling out."

He sat up in bed, put his arms around me, and gave me a firm yet gentle hug. "Are you okay, sweetie?" he asked.

"Not really, but there's not much I can do about it now," I answered.

He kissed me on the cheek and said, "I love you. I'll be waiting tonight, with clippers in hand."

If my hair was coming out, it was going to come out on my terms! So we threw a huge hair-shaving party after work. I wanted to make the whole experience fun, not frightening, for my two-year-old daughter, Nicole. I told her, "The medicine mommy is taking makes my hair fall out. See . . . give it a tug." She reached her tiny hand under the back of my hair and pulled out a big handful of it! Her eyes widened. "Wow, that's neat, Mommy!" she said with a big smile. My best friends and family were all there, too. We drank wine, cooked a big meal, and had a celebration of life. On the outside, I was smiling for the sake of my daughter. On the inside, I was crying, petrified of shaving off all my hair.

Before the scissors came the ribbons. We tied tiny braids in my hair, each one with a pink ribbon on it representing breast cancer. I called them memory locks, and everyone there would cut one off and keep it as a memory of the night. Nicole, with her daddy's help, was the first person to cut one off. She thought it was pretty cool. Then came the clippers. "One, two, three, . . . foooourrrr!" she said, as she buzzed a big strip of hair off my head. Within minutes, the hair that had taken a lifetime to grow was gone. I was bald! "That was fun. Can we do it again tomorrow, Mommy?" Nicole asked.

"No, honey, it's a one-shot deal," I told her.

Then I looked in the mirror. I screamed! Like a child seeing her reflection for the first time, I looked again, and again, and again. That's when something amazing happened. I saw myself! My hair was gone, but I was still there—and still beautiful. What a blessing to have the opportunity to see myself as God sees me! I had to look past the outside and peer deep inside to look at myself as if through his eyes. I realized at that moment my hair had nothing to do with my identity. All the fear and anguish over the prospect of being bald was unfounded and unnecessary. I was beautiful, and I had nothing to be ashamed of!

That's when I made the decision that I would not hide behind my wig. I did wear it on the news, because I didn't want to distract the viewers from what I was saying, but the rest of the time, I walked around bald. If it was cold outside, I put on a baseball hat, but otherwise I walked around bald. My husband shaved his head in support of me and kept his head as bald as mine every day until I finished chemo. You wouldn't believe the looks we got walking around town!

But as I came to terms with being bald, I met so many women who could not. At the oncologist's office, I would meet women who said they admired my boldness to walk around bald—but they could never do it. Some said they had one or two strands of hair left on their head, but they wouldn't cut it, because at least they had hair. Others told me they couldn't bear to see themselves bald and would not take their wigs off in their own homes, even when they were alone. That saddened me terribly. We have so much to worry about, and so much to overcome, that fear of being bald should not be a concern. So I decided to make a statement.

I had already shared with the public my surgery and chemotherapy. Cameras documented my whole battle. On this night, it was time for the third part of my series, how I came to terms with being bald.

So one night, just days after my last chemo treatment, I sat on the set at work without my wig on. The director took the two shot, and there I was, sitting next to my coanchor, balder than a newborn baby. "You see me up here every night, looking healthy and happy," I said. "But this is my reality. I'm bald, and for me, it was the toughest part of my battle against cancer." That was the roll cue to my story on hair loss. I shared with viewers the hair-shaving party and the shock of first seeing myself without hair. "This whole experience has taught me that the prospect of losing my hair was much worse than the reality of it," I said. "Being bald isn't so bad. With that said, I am happy to tell you my hair is growing back as we speak!" We continued with the newscast and the other news of the day. And I continued to anchor the rest of that night without my wig.

The next day, the comment list was once again distributed around the station. Our viewers were very vocal. There were dozens upon dozens of comments, every one of them positive and supportive. My bald head had made a bold point and reached many people in the process. One e-mail made the whole experience worthwhile. A viewer wrote, "Dear Leslie, I just wanted to thank you for representing me up there on the news tonight. I have not been able to come to terms with my hair loss. I haven't been able to walk around my house bald, much less in public. But tonight, after seeing you on the news, I took off my wig and walked down the street to the mailbox. I held my head high and was not ashamed of having no hair on it. Thank you for being you, and for sharing so much with the rest of us."

"Wow!" I thought. "God has used me, and the cancer, to touch other lives."

I was so afraid of going public with my cancer. I was afraid I would be seen as tainted, and it would ruin my career. I was so afraid of losing my hair, afraid I would be ugly and unwanted. With the help and guidance of God, I faced those fears and learned that the old saying is true, "There is nothing to fear, but fear itself."

◈ I HAVE BECOME A stronger, better person because of my battle with cancer, and if given the option, I would never take it back.

God took the cancer and turned it into a multitude of blessings. My career has not been hurt—I was actually promoted at work. My fear of losing my hair was also unfounded. It taught me what I'm made of and gave me a glimpse into my soul. I have become a stronger, better person because of my battle with cancer, and if given the option, I would never take it back.

Today, hair once again sits atop my head. It's short and sassy, and lots of fun! I once again spend time and money coloring it, cutting it, and styling it! But now, when I look in the mirror, I see past the outside and remember the importance of what's inside. What's inside got me through the toughest times of my life and will guide me through the rest of it. Life is precious, and we should all embrace every waking moment! It's a fact of life: We were all born to die. While we have no control over when we'll die, we do have choices about how we will live. I will never again take this fragile gift for granted. I wake up every day and thank God for allowing me one more kiss from my husband, one more hug from my daughter, and one more day of life!

When it's over, it's over. But I won't worry myself about the ending—I will enjoy the journey and see each day as a new beginning.

Sharon Naert

On Their Wings, I Will Find Survival

I've been a flight attendant for American Airlines for 26 years and I love my work! It's been my job to provide care and comfort for passengers, some of whom aren't always pleasant. "Miss, I need a pillow and can't find one!" or "This food tastes funny!" are common complaints. Even though some people aren't agreeable, I try hard to pleasantly provide them with the service I'm paid to give.

During tough flights, I've found a way to help me stay professional, and it has also helped me cope with breast cancer. "No one has control of my feelings without my permission," I've reminded myself many times.

The way I apply it to breast cancer is by realizing this: I have breast cancer; it does not have me. That thought really helps me feel more in control. Cancer may be in my body, but it can't have control over my feelings unless I give it permission. Request denied!

My goal is to remain positive and to make certain that the negative people in my life are no longer part of it. "Are you sure you should go with traditional chemotherapy?" one naysayer asked.

I don't need people second-guessing me. It is hard enough making decisions I think are right for me. If they can't support me, tough! So, as hard as it has been, I have asked unsupportive family members and friends to stop calling me. As you could guess, not everyone has been understanding, but I believe that I've earned the right to take control, like deciding which people going through a revolving door can come into my life and which ones have to stay out of it.

I HAVE BREAST cancer; it does not have me . . . it can't have control over my feelings unless I give it permission.

Another way for me to stay positive is to take walks near my home. I live by Lake Washington in the Seattle area, and when I stroll in the nearby park, my senses stand at attention! I hear the sound of the water washing up on the shore and the leaves crumbling under my brown leather hiking boots. The smell of the leaves and the dirt enriching each other fills me with a sense of renewal.

When I watch the seagulls floating on air over the lake as they screech during their search for dinner, I identify with them. "I know it's a struggle to survive," I think, wondering if they can hear my silent thoughts, as my eyes follow the flight of these white-winged creatures, "and it's a struggle worth experiencing, isn't it?"

Another favorite place for me to reflect is in a tree house 50 feet up in a cedar tree near Mount Rainier. Climbing the 70 wooden steps, arm over arm, step by step to the top, is well worth it. The view of Mount Rainier looming in the distance is nature's reminder of how beautiful and powerful life is and how we must never take it for granted.

I learned that lesson again during my first chemotherapy treatment on September 5, 2001, just six days before the tragedy occurred at the World Trade Center in New York City. Some of my friends and colleagues were killed that day, but they did not die in vain. They reminded me that I have a chance to live and have inspired me to fight as hard as I can to beat breast cancer. They live with me as I grab a tight hold on life and keep them close to my heart.

Alice Keilson Schnaidt

Drumming for Health

T hink of it this way, Alice," my friend Lynn said as she outlined her idea to hold a drumming cere- mony several days before my surgery. "It will be just like gathering your troops before heading into battle." Her suggestion brought to mind age-old images from vin- tage movies: mounted soldiers in gaily colored costumes rid- ing bravely to face the unseen enemy, the solemn-faced drummer boy beating an encouraging tattoo.

I didn't know what to expect. I had never attended a prayer and drumming circle, and one was going to be held in my honor. My hope was that it would give me strength and positive energy for my upcoming mastectomy.

The gathering would be held under the trees in Lynn's leafy backyard. Because I wanted to be surrounded by strong women whom I loved and respected, I invited seven of my closest friends. I hoped that by being around all of them, I would be able to absorb their strength and they would calm my fears.

It was a hot evening in late June when my friends arrived at Lynn's house. Hugging and kissing each one as she walked through the door, I said, "Thank you for coming!" Here they were to lend me their strength. Most of these wonderful women did not know each other. I was their common bond. Almost immediately, I could feel their warmth as I watched how they introduced themselves and heard them talk about their hopes for my successful surgery.

"Why don't each of you take a drum and a candle outside and sit on the blanket on the grass?" Lynn called out.

Drums, big and small, had been carefully arranged on her family room floor, along with some tambourines and seed-filled gourds. Where had she found so many? My friends reached in to pick the ones they preferred, along with the wooden sticks and long-handled wooden spoons to complete their set.

Falling in behind one another, we walked single file through the open sliding-glass door, out to the small backyard, to find a seat on a blue blanket on the soft, dark green grass. Red, pink, and purple flowers framed the yard and seemed to smile at us as we took our positions. The scene was so beautiful. It could have been any outdoor gathering, but tonight it was for me—all for me.

Lynn began the ceremony. "We are gathered here tonight to wish our good friend, Alice, well," Lynn said. "Before we drum our positive thoughts for Alice and ask the universe for her wellness, I would like each one of you to light a candle, share a few thoughts with

THESE PRAYERS formed an inspirational book to which I could turn again and again whenever I felt the need to recapture the strong energy, courage, and love from that extraordinary night.

Alice, and read a prayer or say the blessing you brought with you for her tonight."

I remember how my friend Patti, whom I've known since our sons were in preschool together more than 14 years ago, lit her candle and said, "Alice, you know I am a strong believer in God, and I know he will be on your side during this ordeal."

Everyone who read a prayer that night gave me a copy to take home. Together, these prayers formed an inspirational book to which I could turn again and again whenever I felt the need to recapture the strong energy, courage, and love from that extraordinary night. Here is one of my favorites, from my friend Marcie:

> *Breathe into Me Oh God,*
> *Empty me of angry judgments,*
> *And aching disappointments,*
> *And anxious trying,*
> *And breathe into me*
> *Something like quietness*
> *And confidence,*
> *That the lion and the lamb in me*
> *May lie down together*
> *And be led by a trust*
> *As straightforward as a little child.*
> *Catch my pride and doubt off guard*
> *That, at least for the moment,*
> *I may sense your presence*
> *And your caring,*
> *And be surprised,*
> *by a sudden joy*
> *Rising in me now*
> *To sustain me in the coming then.*

Judie, a neighbor and dear friend, lit a candle and said, "I'll never forget the time you took my two-year-old daughter, Haley, into your home after a car hit our bike at a nearby corner and I had to go to the hospital. You were there for us, and now our entire family wants you to know that we love you and we're praying for you."

Through tears and smiles, we soaked in our love for each other as each friend added more candlelight and positive thoughts to the evening.

Then it was my turn to look each friend in the eye and tell her how much she meant to me. "I love you and I know that I would do anything for you and that you would do anything for me," I remember telling them.

After the last person was addressed, Lynn said, "Everyone, grab your drumsticks and spoons and instruments as we begin to send our healing energy to Alice."

Lynn started with a light boom, boom, boom, boom, and I, along with my friends, joined in as the beat continued, louder and softer and then louder and louder. *Boom, boom, boom, boom, boom, boom, boom, boom.* "God, make me well," I said to myself over and over again. *Boom, boom, boom, boom.* After a few minutes, the drumming stopped. Each of us slowly rose from our places, and I hugged each friend in the circle.

The evening was so loving, powerful, and supportive! With everyone pulling together for me, it made me realize that I was not alone.

As I saw each of my friends fade away through the front door, I felt stronger from their loving thoughts and words and was prepared for the battle ahead of me, knowing my chances of winning had dramatically improved.

Shirley M. Pooley

God, the Unseen Physician

When my friend Pat was passing our swimming pool, her arms laden with flowers, I shouted, "Here I am, in the pool!"

Pat almost stumbled and fell as she tightened her grip on the yellow, orange, and white blossoms. "I thought you just had a mastectomy two weeks ago!" she exclaimed.

"Did you expect me to act like an invalid?" I shot back as I swam triumphantly over to her.

Breast cancer is a life-threatening disease, but it doesn't have to keep a woman down if she relies on, what I call, the Unseen Physician.

The shocking news had been delivered by telephone. When the long-awaited call came, the phone's strident ring jangled my nerves, and my trembling hand clutched the receiver to my ear. "Mrs. Pooley, I have unpleasant news," my doctor said. "Your biopsy revealed breast cancer, but the prognosis is good because it's in the early stage." His voice quickly faded away and was replaced by a secretary's cheerful voice giving me an appointment for the following morning.

I was stunned as I sat at my kitchen table. What had I just heard? Breast cancer? Me?

I remembered the many Sunday services when our minister had prayer requests for the sick and spiritually wounded. On those occasions, I cried silent tears for people who had been stricken with dreaded cancer. Until now, the disease had not afflicted our family, but the big C was happening to me!

Now it was my turn to ask God for his healing help. "Father," I prayed, "take this fear of cancer from me. Let my faith be greater than my fear."

The content and tone of my prayers changed faster than the sky during a summer storm. My mind flashed back to a conversation my friend, Linda, had with God as she lay on the operating table awaiting surgery for a serious liver ailment. Her doctors had done all they could, and she had expected to die. Linda prayed that she should accept God's will, whatever it might be. Shortly after her prayer of surrender to God's will, she began to recover.

Inspired to submit my life and health to God in this manner, I prayed confidently, "God, I don't want the pain of cancer, but if it is your will, I accept it. Please use whatever happens for your purpose and glory."

My ruminations were interrupted by the doorbell. It was Marge and Susan, two friends I had called for support. In an earnest effort, Marge, who had had a mastectomy, lifted her blouse, displaying only one breast. "Look, Cheryl," she said. "I don't even miss mine."

She meant well, but I recoiled in shock and wept. Marge apologized, "I probably shouldn't have done that. I'm used to my scar, but it does take time."

As my friends and I talked, my husband, Gregg, surprised me by arriving home several hours early from a hiking trip. (Susan later confided that she had prayed for his early return.) The sight of him caused me to burst out in tears as I told him the bad news before he even had time to catch his breath.

After my friends left, Gregg and I sat on the couch and embraced, drawing on each other's strength. "I am so sorry you have breast cancer," he said tenderly as he stroked the back of my hair. "We'll get through this together."

The next morning, Gregg and I went to my doctor's office, where Dr. Dixon explained my two treatment choices. "Your first option is a lumpectomy and five weeks of radiation. The other is a simple mastectomy, the complete removal of your right breast. With both surgical procedures, we also remove lymph nodes under the arm to assure the malignancy hasn't spread."

He emphasized that the choice was mine alone. I knew that wasn't really true since I had referred my cancer to the Unseen Physician. My surgery was scheduled to take place in eight days.

Abruptly, Dr. Dixon's voice changed. With a penetrating look, he asked, "How do you feel about losing your breast?"

The question made my head spin. What did that man say? Never before had I been asked such a monumental question. "My 58-year-old body is wearing out and is relatively insignificant compared to the spirit," I responded. "Besides, I believe that God is the great healer."

"I, too, am a believer acting as his instrument," the doctor said. "But remember, you do need surgery."

After the meeting, I returned home, exhausted from trying to absorb all of the new information. Surprisingly, I fell asleep on my double bed only to be awakened by the shrill ring of the telephone. It was Bernadette, a friend who worked as a nurse at a local hospital. As I related my story, the words "breast cancer" didn't sound as strange on my lips.

Bernadette spoke of the numerous mastectomy patients for whom she had cared over the years and how well they recovered and what wonderful lives they have lived. The conversation was so soothing. I felt somewhat like a fighter who had been dazed but was rising before the count of 10. After hanging up the receiver, I looked out the window toward the heavens and spoke, "Father, that call was not a coincidence, was it?"

How closely connected we are with those for whom we pray!

God had brought healing through tender loving care many times during my life, including my battle against alcoholism. Now in the throes of a battle with cancer, I assumed the same blessed medicine would provide the cure.

I had one week to agonize over the choice of surgery. "Please remember me in your prayers," I told my family and my friends at church. It seemed uncanny that two friends reported feeling sympathetic pains in their right breasts while praying for me. How closely connected we are with those for whom we pray!

Hopeful of making an informed decision, I visited with a radiologist, for medical knowledge, as well as with a number of women who had had breast surgery, for moral support and personal observations.

On the morning I was to call my surgeon, a minister friend phoned and suggested I pray in a focused way for guidance in making the right choice. After that conversation, I went to the kitchen counter and picked up a get well card from a large stack. It was from a woman in my Bible class who had personalized Psalm 121 for me. Sitting on the yellow linoleum floor, I meditated on the verses. When I read "The sun will not harm you by day nor the moon at night," I stopped. Here was my answer! The sun won't harm me except by excessive exposure. What was this saying about radiation? A recognition of the danger of radiation led me to believe God had provided the answer.

I called the doctor and told him to perform a mastectomy. I slept peacefully that night. The surgery the following afternoon went smoothly, and I took only two pain pills. It was a significant victory for an addictive person like me. Prayer rather than pills was my sedative. Prayer allayed my fears and eased the pain.

One morning while I was convalescing, Gregg asked how I was feeling. Tears trickled down my cheeks as I told him that I felt depressed. My husband took me by the hand, seating me in his oversized, brown wooden rocking chair, and turned on the stereo. A beautiful praise hymn filled the room. Soon my spirit was soaring with the music. With a loving husband like mine, it is difficult to stay down in the dumps. I was also deluged with flowers, phone calls, cards, and visits from my family and friends. Love came in many forms from the Divine Healer.

At first, I felt self-conscious about my flat chest, but this attitude was short-lived. The doctor explained that breast reconstruction was available six months after surgery, but I never seriously considered it. I believe God gave women breasts for nursing babies, not to flaunt and attract men. My mothering days were long past. I opted for a prosthesis. My self-consciousness disappeared when Gregg showed me that he still found me desirable.

Affirmations came from everyone. Our daughter works as a visiting nurse with the terminally ill. When I shared with her my amazement at the affection I was receiving, she gave me another gift. "Mom, you are only reaping what you have sown in the past."

As I look back on my experience, I understand that when I prayed for God's will to be done, his treatment plan unfolded. Dr. Dixon was his assistant, as were my family and friends who walked through those frightening weeks with me.

Six weeks have passed since my surgery, and I have resumed all normal activities. By swimming daily, I have regained complete use of my arm. Greatest of all, the Unseen Physician brought me safely through, healing my body and spirit, and once again renewed my faith.

A New Me

I'm coming to terms with a new me.

It's been two months since my mastectomy. Two months not of pain, but of discomfort, restrained movements, trying to find comfortable positions for my body, stuffing brassieres with some sort of filling and praying everything stays in the right place.

Before that was the fear. Fear of the knife, but most of all, fear of the word: cancer. My sister had just died of it. She was cremated and her remains were scattered in the desert near her home.

Was this to be the end for me? Would I never see my youngest son marry, father children? Would I never share the holidays with friends again? Would I lose the joy of living, being a part of this beautiful world?

I didn't know.

I didn't know until a week after the surgery when my doctor told me he thought they'd gotten all the cancer, the lymph nodes were negative, and tests showed the cancer was not aggressive. Essentially, he said: You can get on with your life. No radiation. No chemotherapy. The only postsurgical treatment was a twice-daily tamoxifen pill to ward off recurring cancer.

So I was joyful in response, impulsively climbing on my tiptoes to throw a bear hug around my very professional surgeon, who tolerated my rapture with an enigmatic smile. I went home feeling relief that now I could make plans, care for my home, travel again, be there for my family.

But relief is not all of it. First came the business of learning to live in a changed body. Exercising an arm that would rather not move. Lying in bed and trying to decide if sleep would come as you lay on your side (as you always slept before) or on your back (relieving stress on that arm). Trying to get into clothing with an arm that just couldn't twist that way without excruciating pain. Exercising (as directed) and wondering if it would hurt too much to do those reaches or if you dare stretch a little farther.

ᑫᗺᒐ *ONCE YOU'VE AC-cepted all that, you can relish the rest and let the marks on the wall tell a story of the positive joys of existence.*

You see, it just didn't feel like me anymore. I wasn't predictable. I had always been predictable. I swam, hiked, gardened, and always had the feeling that my body could do just about anything I wanted it to. Not as much as when I was 10 and, if I was running as fast as I could, I knew I could always run a little faster. I gave up that feeling long ago. But my body usually performed on order.

Now I didn't know about my body. Maybe it could do that and maybe it couldn't. I made black marks on the white wall to demonstrate how high my fingers could go, and the white wall showed marks moving up only slowly, or sometimes not at all.

There were moments of triumph when the fingers crept higher, but of resignation, too, when they just couldn't make another fraction of an inch.

A mastectomy is a giant leap on the road to aging. I was well aware I was traveling down that road, but it actually didn't feel real to me before. Now sometimes I feel ancient. The body betrayal of poor balance, stiff limbs, mottled skin confronts me and leaves me no excuses. I'm getting old. One of the insults life hands you is an aging body.

But somehow, once you've accepted it—the prosthesis problems, the lopsided feeling in the shower, the last ache of a muscle that works reluctantly—once you've accepted all that, you can relish the rest and let the marks on the wall tell a story of the positive joys of existence.

The new me is so glad to be among the living.

Becky Richards, R.N.

Never Say Never

I'm a recovery room care nurse. You've probably seen those images on the TV show *ER* when patients are whisked on a gurney into the emergency room for treatment. I've seen how patients' families sob as they've watched terminally ill loved ones endure nurses poking them with needles, inserting intravenous tubes, and suctioning fluids from their throats.

From watching those scenes, I made a pact with myself. If cancer ever invaded my body, I'd never get surgery or chemotherapy. I couldn't handle the thought of my husband, son, or daughter watching me suffer. The quality of life is better than quantity of life, I decided. There was no way I was going to alter what time I had left on earth by spending it on surgery and chemotherapy, I promised myself.

But when I was diagnosed with breast cancer, those thoughts quickly went out the window. You know why? Because I overlooked the fact that I have only one life, and whatever that life is, I want it and I'll fight for it!

Instead of isolating myself, I decided to take my family and friends on the journey with me by sharing my thoughts from diagnosis to surgery to chemotherapy. They were all so concerned about me and wanted to know the details, so I sent them a group letter about each step along the way.

I HAVE ONLY ONE life, and whatever that life is, I want it and I'll fight for it!

My life was one thing; my hair, on the other hand, posed one of my biggest challenges. Chemotherapy robbed me of my beautiful, thick, blond shoulder-length hair. About two weeks after my first treatment, my scalp was itchy, and as I scratched, I could feel strands of hair wrapping tightly around my fingers. It was frightening and disgusting to see how much came off of my head!

Did I have the courage to go through this every day? To watch slowly as my lovely hair left me? Nope. I called my friend Christy, who's a hairdresser. "I think it's time to shave my head," I told her.

Now this was not an act I could endure in a public beauty shop. Christy suggested her kitchen. I could feel her hands and eyes examining my head. "Let's cut it short instead of shaving it," she said. "Don't be in such a hurry to shave it!"

I agreed and after the last tress fell onto her linoleum floor, Christy said, "This will buy you a few days. It looks real different, so don't be too surprised when you go into the bathroom and take a look."

Walking down her familiar hallway, I felt strong and determined. When I entered the bathroom and caught sight of the unfamiliar face in mirror, it hit me. "I can't get off this roller coaster because I'm strapped in!" I thought.

Christy heard my muffled sobs and quickly came to my side. Then I broke down and cried in my friend's arms. Christy is 14 years younger than I am, and it was as if our roles were reversed. I'd always been there for her and her family. Now she was mothering me. Christy's kids had never seen me so sad. Twelve-year-old Andrea, nine-year-old Jake, and two-year-old Zach were in the other room when my hair was cut, but as their mom and I were locked in a tearful hug, I could feel their arms and bodies hugging my legs and patting my back. Christy said, "Becky, you are the strongest person I know! It's about time you cried!"

A week after that, I was bald. I didn't mind it so much at home, but when I went out in public, it was another story. No one knew, unless I told them, about my not having breasts. However, when people saw me without any hair on my head, I became an open target for questions that I may or may not have been prepared to answer, like the time I ran into an old friend who was a grocery store checker. As Debbie pulled my cart forward, she looked up with surprise. She lightly lifted my blue baseball hat and said, "Becky, what has happened to you?"

"I have breast cancer," I blurted out, so loudly that everyone within earshot could hear. Debbie hugged me, as the strangers in line dabbed their eyes. They weren't the only ones crying. "I'm doing okay," I reassured her through my tears. "I'm not dying from this!"

I wanted to crack a joke and say something like, "I got a boob job for life, and look at how much money I'm saving on shampoo."

That incident taught me a lesson. People need to know about breast cancer, and it's important to tell them you don't have to die from it. It can actually be a blessing, because unlike people who are killed or maimed by a drunk driver in a car accident and who may never have told their loved ones how much they cared, breast cancer reminds you to reexamine your life and to make the most of it.

Why me? Why you? I have been asked so many times why this has happened to me and why that has happened to others. I do not have the answer, of course. But what I do know is that none of us has any guarantees in life. What I do see is an opportunity. It's to make my life count in an intense way.

JoAnne Gray George

Breast Cancer Is Just Another Speed Bump

Maybe if I ignore this, it will go away. That's what I thought as I stepped from the shower after finding a walnut-sized lump under my right breast.

My husband and I were preparing to leave the next day on a much-needed vacation to Hawaii, and I promised myself if the lump was still there when we returned in 10 days, I would call the doctor.

There's no need to worry, I told myself. How serious could it be? I had a mammogram three months earlier and it wasn't there then . . . or was it?

I had had numerous cysts in the past, so it probably was just another one . . . or was it?

Wanting so much for our vacation to be a renewal of our commitment to each other, I didn't mention a word to my husband.

When we returned home, the lump was still there, and I called the doctor, who saw me immediately. Tests were conducted in no time, and after a diagnostic mammogram and an ultrasound, the verdict was clear by the look on the radiologist's face. His words reinforced it. "Whatever this thing is," he said, "it has to come out."

It was back to my doctor in the afternoon, and as I waited endlessly for my turn, I noticed things I would never have paid attention to under normal circumstances: scattered magazines, leaflet holders that needed filling, a large brown spider walking up the wall as it quickly crept toward a white cabinet filled with medical supplies. Usually, I would have found something to use to dispose of that spider, but suddenly, I felt myself mesmerized as I wondered, "Is that spider going to outlive me?"

The doctor finally appeared, and I could see by his worried face that he was struggling to find the right words to tell me what I obviously did not want to hear. Quietly and gently, he said, "I'm sorry, but your lump has all the indications of being malignant. I strongly suggest that you have a mastectomy and forget about radiation because it will burn your skin."

His words confused me. Why would I want to trade a sunburn for a breast? "Give me a few days to think about it," I told the doctor. "I need some time to make a decision before I see the surgeon."

It all seemed so surreal to me. I am a vice president at our community hospital and raised the funds for an outpatient cancer center two years earlier. As I stared at the brass-framed picture of the cancer center on my office wall, I thought, "I never dreamed I'd become one of your patients."

Within a few days, I had to make up my mind about how doctors would deal with my cancer. Writing is a very important part of my life, and I listed the pros and cons on a piece of paper. With each word I wrote, I could feel some anxiety leave my body as my brain took over the process of decision making. I put a lumpectomy in the pro column opposite a mastectomy in the con column. To me, the lumpectomy was the clear choice, because unlike the mastectomy, it required minor surgery, it would save my breast, and there wouldn't be a need for reconstruction.

The lumpectomy and node dissection confirmed cancer, and my oncologist prescribed chemotherapy followed by radiation. There were days in the next few months that I was so tired, I couldn't put one foot in front of the other, but I managed to go to work almost every day. Once I was so tired that I went to bed for 24 hours. It was so rejuvenating that I was able to return to my normal schedule the next day.

I COULD WHINE about my health and cry about losing my hair, or I could continue living my life to the best of my ability and truly believe that cancer was not going to defeat me.

Early on in my treatment, I decided that I had two choices. I could take a leave of absence from work, whine about my health and cry about losing my hair as I worried about dying, or I could continue living my life to the best of my ability, buy a wig, put on a happy face no matter what, and truly believe that cancer was *not* going to defeat me. It was just another speed bump in the road of life.

My positive attitude helped two years later when breast cancer was diagnosed on the left side. At first, I was afraid that I was to blame for starting the cycle of pain all over again for everyone in my family. After all, we had been through so much already with my cancer, and with my mother being diagnosed with terminal cancer as well as a cancer diagnosis for my sister and brother-in-law. All of the illnesses were devastating to our family, and a psycho-oncology therapist helped me take the guilt burden off of my shoulders and continued to counsel me during the treatment that followed.

What also helped was the power of prayer. I had been raised a Catholic, but after a painful divorce, I turned away from structured religion. However, I found that I had never turned away from God or from finding a sense of peace through prayer during troubled times.

When I found my rosary tucked away in a blue velvet box in the back of my dresser drawer, I held it up to the light to look at the creamy pearl and gold filigree beads. As I held the beads in my hands, my eyes filled with tears, thankful for the reconnection with God and the hope they brought to me.

What does the future hold for me? Will my body continue to fight cancer? I honestly don't know. The one thing I am certain of is that breast cancer has been a challenge to my health, but it will never have the ability to take away what is dear to me, including the love and support of my family and friends and, most of all, my belief in God's plan for my life.

Mary M. Borel

Listen to Your Body

When I was a nurse back in the early 1970s in the small town of Independence, Kansas, doctors were placed on such a high pedestal that when they came to the nurses' station, we ladies, dressed in our starched white dresses and caps, would automatically stand up to greet them and say, "Good afternoon [or, Good evening], doctor," depending on the time of day. We respected them for the knowledge they had, and we knew where our places were when it came to delivering medical care.

So when my family doctor of many years told me not to worry about the itchy and hardened nipple on my left breast, I assumed he knew a lot more than I did and that he had to be right. I was a mother of five children under the age of 16, and I was much too busy raising them and working a part-time job to worry about second-guessing a doctor. (Looking back now, I can't help but think, "God, Almighty, I was stupid!")

That nipple bothered me for a good year. I did routine monthly breast self-exams, never felt any lumps or anything, and thought, "This will just go away or I'll just have to learn to live with it."

It wasn't until I was on duty at the local hospital when I discovered that there really was something to worry about. A friend who was in the hospital for an impending hysterectomy asked me to look up something in a medical book concerning her condition. During my break, I went to the hospital's library. As I scanned rows and rows of medical books, my eyes zeroed in on a large, reddish purple gynecological surgery volume. I quickly found the article my friend needed, and then my eyes caught sight of a heading on the same page, "Paget's Disease." I glanced at it in disbelief. It included a complete description of an itching, burning, hardening nipple!

The next day I went back to my doctor and asked for a biopsy and once again listened to him tell me, "Oh, Mary, I don't think so, but if it will you make you feel better . . ."

You've probably guessed by now that the biopsy came back positive for cancer. The surgeon delivered the bad news two days later, while I was working at the hospital's nursing station, filling in a patient's chart. "I've talked this over with your family physician, and we've decided that a lumpectomy would be the best, and we'll operate on Monday," the surgeon said.

THE CANCER DIAGnosis was made when I was 48 years old. I'm happy and proud to tell you that I'm 76 years old now and healthy as a horse!

"Oh, no you won't!" I responded with anger and a newfound sense of control. I knew where my place was, all right. It was advocating for me. "You'll send me to Wichita for the surgery," I said.

Did he really think that after my doctor let this thing live in my body for a year that I'd trust him to take it out? (Maybe I wasn't so stupid, after all!)

The rest is history. The surgeon in Wichita decided against a lumpectomy and in favor of a modified radical mastectomy, and it appears his decision was right.

The cancer diagnosis was made when I was 48 years old. I'm happy and proud to tell you that I'm 76 years old now and healthy as a horse! I have done a lot of living and have learned some lessons the hard way.

Please take the advice that I share with my children and grandchildren. Listen to your body, not only to the doctors who treat you. Bring up any questions or concerns you have, and if your physician pooh-poohs them, find someone else to treat you. Don't just accept an "It's okay" statement. It's up to you to be sure it is okay.

Miss Understood: From Outer Beauty to Inner Strength

When I was in seventh grade, living in Chicago, Illinois, my friend Judy Plate and I went into the school bathroom and stuffed our bras with scratchy toilet paper. We giggled with excitement as we transformed ourselves from being flat as a board to, in our eyes, curvaceous as a voluptuous movie star. We flung open the bathroom door with a sense of "Here we come, world," and we were filled with artificially fed confidence as our chests reached places before the rest of our bodies did. The problem was, I hadn't realized that my bra was totally lopsided and you could see the crinkles through my shirt. One look, and the other kids started pointing and snickering and the teasing didn't stop for years.

Unfortunately, being ridiculed was nothing new to me. By the time I was 12, I was 5 feet 8 inches tall and weighed 100 pounds—stick thin, flat chested, and not a curve in sight, and you better believe I heard about it . . . often!

"Are you a girl or a boy?" I was often asked. Other hurtful comments included: "Stand sideways and stick out your tongue—you'll look like a zipper" and "Do you model for a match factory?"

After spending an agonizing childhood being kidded about how I looked, I was able to turn that "disability" into a glamorous, exciting, and lucrative modeling and acting career—a career that, I believe, ended up saving my life. Becoming a model and an actress made me feel like I had been transformed from an ugly ducking into a beautiful swan.

You may have seen me as a mom in a famous Johnson & Johnson baby shampoo commercial in which I ran through a field in slow motion with my long, shiny blond hair bouncing on and off of my shoulders. I starred in other national television commercials, pushing products like Close-Up toothpaste, Maybelline makeup, and Sara Lee baked goods.

In my career, I was the spokesperson for well over 2,000 national television commercials, appeared in every major fashion magazine, played in 26 theater productions, had a role in four films, hosted two talk shows, starred in 10 years of soap operas, appeared in television shows like *The Love Boat, Different Strokes,* and *Love American Style,* and was an entertainment editor for *Inside Edition.*

In 1979, I met my husband, Steve, who owned a famous New York restaurant, Herlihy's (his family name). A year and a half after our son, Logan, was born, I found a lump the size of a marble on my left breast. I immediately called a doctor friend of mine, who suggested it was a blocked milk gland since I had recently finished breast-feeding. I was relieved when a mammogram showed nothing, confirming my friend's guess. "It will disappear eventually," I told myself.

A year later, when I was 43, the lump was still there, and doctors said it would have to be removed before I could have breast implants. I had wanted those implants so badly because I knew they would help me look better in the bathing suits I was modeling while working and living in Fort Lauderdale, Florida. The surgeon knew as soon as he saw the lump that it was a cancerous tumor, and when I awoke from the anesthetic, the surgeon said, "We'll have to hold off on those implants. I'm sorry, but you have cancer and we'll have to perform a radical mastectomy very soon."

How could this be? I had a mammogram and it showed nothing. I was livid but knew that anger was a waste of my energy. (If I had to do it over, I would have insisted the doctor do an aspiration the first day I went to my gynecologist.)

The next few weeks seemed like a blur, and my focus was not on the camera but on getting well. On October 1, 1990, I had the surgery and reconstruction after six months of chemotherapy. My long, beautiful blond hair disappeared, and the only bookings I got were doctor appointments. But I didn't miss the glamour of my career. What I really missed was being able to hug my two-year-old son, Logan, and four-and-a-half-year-old daughter, Taylor, and having the energy to chase them around the house like I did before the diagnosis. Logan and Taylor were so sweet during my recovery! They would sit with me on my king-sized bed and "read" me stories, use their crayons to make me get well cards, carry food on a tray with their little hands, rub my feet, and be quiet when I needed to sleep while going through chemotherapy. "Sssh! Mommy needs to sleep," I once heard Taylor tell her little brother outside my bedroom door, peeking at me through the crack.

My husband, Steve, also proved that he loved me for who I am and not what I look like. Steve made love to me the night I came home from the hospital. Any second thoughts I had about my desirability were immediately erased. It was the most incredible experience of our marriage! Steve held me and cooed in my ear and stroked my hair and kissed away my tears. He whispered things about loving me, not my boobs, and how I filled his life and completed him. His tenderness and love gave me such strength and fortitude! How did I ever get so lucky and blessed?

Lessons of love were also taught by my friends, who called and wrote supportive letters from all over the country when they found out the news. One high school friend flew to Florida from Cincinnati to hang out with me for four days. She brought old yearbooks and we laughed and reminisced as we carefully scanned each page and face. I felt cleansed and healed from that time together. What also helped was the "victory list" she had me write of all the things I had accomplished so far in my life. "Wow! I have done a lot!" I thought, looking at the long list on yellow tablet paper.

> *What also helped was the "victory list" she had me write of all the things I had accomplished so far in my life.*

My career wasn't ruined. By the time I had been diagnosed with cancer, I really had done it all. There wasn't much about show business that excited me anymore. It was time to be a mom, focus on my family, get closer to God, and find my purpose. I finally believed that I deserved happiness and realized that success is not equated with money.

Now when I look at fashion magazines, I realize that I had a fabulous experience that molded me into who I am today. By focusing on my outsides and obsessing about my looks, I had nowhere else to look but inside.

All of that soul-searching and battling hard against breast cancer have helped me in the job I've been doing for the last eight years as a corporate trainer. I can share funny and touching stories from my "previous life" as I give motivational speeches to people who want to improve their personal and professional lives.

In addition to my part-time work, I'm a college student again, working toward a bachelor's degree in Applied Behavioral Science. Am I trying to look good to others on the outside again? No way! I'm doing it for me. I'm enjoying my full life—my husband, children, and work. It's a great life, which I embrace one day at a time. Why? Well, as they say in the commercials, "Because I'm worth it!"

Do Unto Others

As I neared the end of chemotherapy, the simplest words filled me with emotion. Bad news could knock me flat, and good news made me giddy with laughter. Eight months ago, when I heard the diagnosis "cancer" and went through a lumpectomy and then a second surgery to take out a larger, clean margin around the tumor site, I avoided talking about it. Silence was my way of coping. I worked hard not to describe the experience, even to myself. As I approach radiation therapy, which starts next week, I have learned a valuable lesson: that the right words are the best possible therapy I can prescribe for myself.

The loss of my hair was the catalyst I needed to bring me around. Looking at my naked head in the mirror made it impossible to practice avoidance. Gazing at a few remaining wisps of my frosted hair sticking out in totally random, strangely defiant angles, the stoic part of me withered. My eyes, nose, and mouth took on huge proportions and stood out vengefully. Hair softens the flaws, especially in my case.

Without it, I had no distractions and few pretenses. Even on the days I felt reasonably good, my reflection provided a constant reminder of how little I could do to control this disease.

Feelings of helplessness accompanied me when I went to look for a wig. My husband encouraged me to drive from our hometown of Naperville, Illinois, toward the city of Chicago to a shop that came highly recommended. The salesperson, barely 5 feet tall, struck me as someone's grandmother trapped in a teenager's body. Many women her age, who are as thin and small-boned as she, have started to stoop over. Not June. She stood straight and ready for anything. I don't remember what she said in the way of greeting. I was practicing denial and wanted to be anywhere else but there. But I do remember that she escorted me to a private room and then leaned in close, invading my space. "Talk to me," she said. As if nothing could be more natural than confiding in a stranger.

It is neither easy or natural for me to open up like that. "I'm a chemotherapy patient, and I need a wig," I muttered.

June's eyes narrowed as if she were gently scolding her grandson. "We don't use the word *wig* here. We like to call it your *new hair*."

For the next two hours, as I sat at a gray vanity facing a rectangular mirror, we looked at my changing reflection while June fitted my head with different styles of new hair, all close to the same frosted blond color I normally wore. June's hands kept moving, brushing, combing, and carefully positioning strands of new hair on my head. Her attention and encouragement told me, "This is important, and so are you."

But vastly more valuable than making sure I looked my best, she gradually helped me talk about what I was facing.

After 40 years in the business, she had stored up a lifetime of knowledge and wanted to hear about things no one except my husband thought to ask. She quizzed me about the pathology of my tumor, about treatment plans, and I found myself telling her all the things that I had bottled up inside. In fact, she spent 80 percent of her time just talking to me and only about 20 percent trying to sell her wares.

Eventually, we got serious about the reason for my visit. After trying on several different styles, June asked, "What do you think of this one?"

"I don't know," I said. "I'd like to try a red one since a number of family members are redheads."

Before I could say anything else, June quickly disappeared to return with a short, wispy paprika-red wig . . . I mean, hair.

She stretched it over my scalp, and you know what? I have the right complexion to go with red hair. It looked like it was made just for me! One of those giddy smiles I cannot control spread across my face and stayed there for hours.

> *Her careful use of words taught me a valuable lesson—the way we describe life's obstacles makes them either impossible or easier to overcome.*

But June sent me away with more than new hair. She also gave me a new attitude. Her careful use of words taught me a valuable lesson—the way we describe life's obstacles makes them either impossible or easier to overcome.

Now when I look in the mirror—whether I see a redhead or bald dome—I'm reminded of June's kindness. Even if I can't control the cancer, I'm not helpless. I can do positive things and pass along encouraging words and ideas to others. Maybe that's one of the reasons why I decided to participate in a clinical trial for a drug called herceptin, an antibody agent used for certain types of advanced cancers.

If it weren't for the women before me who underwent lumpectomies combined with radiation to test their effectiveness, I wouldn't have had the benefit of the treatment I'm using. If it weren't for these brave souls, our only option today might still be radical mastectomies. And what about the women who took experimental drugs now regularly used to treat breast cancer? How could I turn my back on future breast cancer patients? Now it's my turn to step forward and help. Who knows? If the trial proves this antibody to be effective for stage 2 cancers, I may be helping myself as well as my three sisters and four nieces, not to mention countless women I will never know, who share a common bond with me.

Eight months ago, breast cancer felt like a lonely and isolating experience. I knew the moment the doctor described the clinical trial that I wanted to help researchers tame this disease. That decision helped immensely, but focusing on the long term did less than I thought it would. On the bad days, it wasn't the kind of consolation I craved. Thank heaven for June, who taught that the reflection in the mirror didn't define my situation—I did. A willingness to talk, searching for the right words if you have to, makes all the difference in the world. And because of her and generous people like her along the way, I've learned how to connect to others in many positive ways.

Reach Out and Touch Someone

ello?" The voice on the telephone sounded low and timid. It reflected all the uncertainty, fear, and sadness that one might expect from a person who had been diagnosed with cancer. The very timbre of Kathy's voice was dark and melancholy.

"Hello, Kathy," I said warmly. "My name is Barbara, and I am a volunteer with Reach to Recovery. Your doctor gave me your name, and I would like to find a time to visit with you. I am a breast cancer survivor, and I have some gifts for you."

"Oh, thank you!" Some life came back into her voice. "Can you come tomorrow?"

We exchanged information about time and driving directions, and I assured Kathy that I would be happy to visit with her and to answer any questions that I could. And if I couldn't answer them, I could help her find the best source of information.

Reach to Recovery is a volunteer organization sponsored by the American Cancer Society. All the volunteers are breast cancer survivors who reach out and touch others who have been diagnosed. Remembering the dark and depressing time of our treatments allows us to create a bond with newly diagnosed patients.

As I prepared for my visit to see Kathy, I remembered my own Reach to Recovery visit. In January 1997, I lay in a hospital bed in Brussels, Belgium, feeling very sorry for myself. Just before Christmas, I had been diagnosed with breast cancer. The excitement and bright lights of the holiday season had given way to dull, gray days and sad, terrifying nights. The darkness seemed to take over any feelings of hope.

My husband and I kept that dreadful secret to ourselves through the holidays, not wanting to upset our family. We used that time to read as much as we could find about breast cancer. It was daunting to think about having a life-threatening disease and being treated for it in a foreign country. Nonetheless, January found me in a cancer hospital having a mastectomy.

I had read about Reach to Recovery and about how volunteers answer nonmedical questions, teach exercises to regain the use of arms where lymph nodes have been removed, and provide a temporary prosthesis to wear until the surgical healing allows a permanent prosthesis. It was exactly what I needed, but what was I to do in a foreign country without the American Cancer Society? I craved the comfort of a conversation with a woman who had been through what I now faced.

The prosthesis—now, that worried me. What would I do to look normal? How could I hide my lopsidedness? My 16-year-old daughter already worried that her friends might talk about my breast—a no-no for adolescents. On the night of my release from the hospital, we were hosting a preparty for the winter formal. Ashley and a dozen of her friends would show up in party finery, and she would be so embarrassed if her mom appeared breastless.

As I lay there, feeling sorry for myself, with a single tear escaping onto the pillow, I wondered for the first time why I had not returned to the United States for my treatment. The answer was simple. I wanted my family around me, and my family was in Belgium. But Reach to Recovery wasn't in Belgium, and how would I get a prosthesis to see me through my surgical healing?

While I wallowed in self-pity, I must have drifted off. I awakened to find a guest in my hospital room, a lovely woman whom I did not know. An attractive, middle-aged woman, she was wearing a clinging red sweater that accentuated her shape. "Would I ever wear something like that again?" I wondered.

Before I could become more depressed at that thought, my guest, Madame Carstairs, explained in flawless English, "Hello, Barbara. I am a volunteer with Vivre Comme Avant. I know you are an American, so perhaps you have heard of our organization in your country. It is called Reach to Recovery. Here it means 'to live as before.'"

My mind was spinning. If Madame Carstairs was a Reach to Recovery volunteer, then she, too, must be a breast cancer survivor. She continued, "I had the same surgery you have just had. You see, I am recovered and healthy, and you will be, too."

Madame Carstairs provided information about cancer and healing. "I can help you when you are ready to buy a prosthesis or if you need a wig," she added. But most important, this lovely woman brought a temporary prosthesis. She would save me from the embarrassment of going home with half a flat chest. With this gift, the tears flowed in gratitude. This lovely woman answered my prayers, lifted my spirits, and solved my problem. She pinned the prosthesis inside my bra before she left me, and I gushed out my thanks.

As I drove to Kathy's home to make my first Reach to Recovery visit, I mentally thanked Madame Carstairs again and recalled the joy that walked into my room with her visit.

I rang the doorbell, feeling unsure about what to expect and even a little nervous. Kathy answered the door and invited me in. The house was as dark as the mood. Kathy sat huddled on a brown sofa, hugging a pillow under her arm and spreading an afghan over her legs. The curtains were closed, and the air seemed oppressive. I took a deep breath and reminded myself that I brought comfort and hope.

"How are you feeling, Kathy?" I began.

"I guess I feel a little better each day," she responded listlessly. "My surgery was five days ago. I live alone, and my daughters come to help me when they get off work in the afternoons."

No wonder she was sad. Cancer is a frightening disease to go through alone. I was even more determined to cheer her up. "I have brought you some gifts from the American Cancer Society. Shall I explain what I have here?"

As I went through the various pamphlets about breast cancer, treatment, recovery, and support, Kathy perked up. It was difficult to see the pamphlets, so I suggested that I open the curtains. With the sun pouring in, the room looked brighter and more cheery. Kathy herself warmed up a bit as she heard about support programs that were available in the community.

"Now, Kathy, I would like to demonstrate some exercises for you. I don't want you to do them yet. You have to wait until you get your stitches out and the doctor says you may exercise. At that time, you will regain the mobility in your arm by doing these exercises."

I faced a nearby wall and put both of my hands up against it. "When you're ready, Kathy," I said looking back at her over my right shoulder, "you will use your fingers to walk up the wall as high as they can go. It can be painful, at first, but as your arms gain strength, the pain will subside, and the higher your fingers will be able to climb."

I also showed Kathy how to use a palm-sized soft ball. "Squeezing it helps build your strength and it relieves stress," I explained.

My other exercise gift was a pulley made of 5 to 6 feet of rope with handles on each end. I showed Kathy how the pulley worked to strengthen her arms. I laughed at the strange position I was in. Even Kathy laughed, saying I looked like a dressed-up aerobics instructor. Her laughter sounded great! It lightened up the visit and made us feel like old friends.

Finally, I pulled the temporary, beige, fiber-filled prosthesis out of the gift bag. "Kathy, you can pin this into your bra and wear it until you are healed enough to be fitted for a permanent prosthesis. If it is too big, just pull out some of the stuffing. If it is too small, you can use some of the extra fiberfill that is in this bag. The form is even washable in your washing machine."

By the time the visit ended, Kathy and I were friends. The common bond of breast cancer allowed us to talk about intimate and important subjects on our first meeting, like worrying about our daughters getting breast cancer, too, about feeling attractive, and about going into menopause. I gave Kathy my telephone number, and I told her I would call her again. I was so happy that I had brightened her home and her day, even for a short time.

As I made more visits to "sisters" in the breast cancer sorority, I met many different types of women. Every woman felt frightened, but each approached the journey ahead with different individual concerns and needs. Sometimes we could laugh together; sometimes we cried together. Some women were in denial and others were upbeat about winning the battle against breast cancer. With every visit, my own healing continued. By reaching out to others, my own fears subsided because the talking helped chase away some of the fears of the unknown.

Cancer does not end when the treatment finishes. Cancer remains a part of one's life forever. Every time I reach out and touch someone, I feel grateful that I traveled the path of cancer so that I can spread the hope of recovery and the joy of living another day.

The second anniversary of my cancer diagnosis brought a Christmas of family celebration and happy times, very different from the Christmas of two years before when my husband and I kept the terrifying cancer secret to ourselves. On Christmas evening, I received a special phone call from a young woman whom I had visited for Reach to Recovery. Despite her difficult experience with a double mastectomy, she did not want Christmas day to pass without expressing how glad she felt to be alive.

> *Reach out and touch someone, and the healing continues.*

"How can I ever thank you enough, a person I didn't even know yet who cared enough to help me, to visit and to pray for me?" she asked.

"It was my pleasure," I told her. "No thanks are necessary!"

Her phone call completed an already joyful day.

For several years, I kept the prosthesis that my guardian angel, Madame Carstairs, had given me. It is a little beige sac filled with fiberfill. I wore that soft prosthesis for months after my surgery, long after I could have been fitted for a permanent prosthesis. It carried with it the symbolism of love and concern from another human being. And it served the purpose well.

Nearing my fifth anniversary of cancer treatment, I received a call from a friend. She told me the bad news that she was scheduled to have a mastectomy and she was agonizing over the decision about whether to have reconstruction.

Without a moment's hesitation, I suggested, "Come over on Saturday. I will show you all the mastectomy supplies I have, explain how they are used, and I will even show you my scar." When I hung up the phone, I wondered if my offer was appropriate, but my friend accepted the invitation.

Our visit together demystified the prospect of having a mastectomy and helped her make her own personal decision about treatment. On an impulse, I suggested, "If you want to take this temporary prosthesis, you are more than welcome. It is great to wear home from the hospital, and you can use it until you are healed enough for a permanent prosthesis."

My friend was thrilled to have her problem solved. And my spirits soared to think that I might be her guardian angel by making this simple gift. Reach out and touch someone, and the healing continues.

You Gotta Have Friends

My friends and family have been a source of strength and support throughout my ordeal with breast cancer. During the Christmas holiday in 2000, I went home to Salem, Oregon, from a village in Alaska where I had been teaching elementary school children. That's when I found out that I had breast cancer. From diagnosis on December 26, 2000, to my first round of chemotherapy on December 29 to reduce the tumor before my scheduled modified radical mastectomy, friends and family were with me at the doctors' offices, at the hospital, and at home. They shared the sad news with me when a bone scan showed that cancer had metastasized to the hipbones, meaning I was in stage 4 at the age of 63. And they shared my joy when, six months later, a bone scan showed no new lesions and that the existing ones were less conspicuous.

I'll never forget the Time for Healing Party we shared on New Year's Eve, just days after my first chemotherapy treatment. There were nine of us, including me, and each one of my friends wrote words of encouragement on separate pieces of white rectangular paper. The papers were rolled up and placed into a glass jar with a rainbow of colored ribbons taped to the top. Those notes were such a source of strength and encouragement to me; I think I read each and every one of them twice until surgery.

Besides writing notes, my friends had researched the healing customs of different cultures, and we practiced some of them. For example, each of us threw a small loaf of French bread at a door, and we banged on oatmeal boxes and pots and pans to drive away evil spirits. We also randomly chose a card from a deck of angel cards, reading aloud different inspirational messages of positive energy about dealing with life's challenges.

Four of these wonderful ladies, all teachers, insisted on coming with me to the hospital when I went to have surgery. They were with me up until the time I was taken into the operating room. I was fortunate, too, when my friends accompanied me to my first chemo treatment. They brought lunches and we all ate and visited while I entered a new phase of fighting cancer. I have to say, it was such a glorious feeling and such a burden off my shoulders when I lost the breast and got rid of that tumor! I'm so thankful to have my feet, hands, hearing, and eyesight. I certainly didn't need the breast.

About the time I began radiation, a friend gave me Hope, the Breast Cancer Research bear, and she attended my radiation sessions with me. Another friend gave me Strength, the Avon cancer bear, and a support group friend presented me with Courage, a Susan Komen teddy bear. The stuffed trio has joined me at my ever-helpful support group meetings and at my monthly pamidronate (bone strengthener) treatments. I can hug them if I need to, or I can pose them on a table so I can look at them and feel the closeness of the friends who gave them to me. (Another friend quilted a beautiful pillow for me with a picture on the front of me at the finish line of a race holding our group's medals. I sleep with that pillow every night and take it on trips.)

What also helped me with the healing process was keeping busy. I was fortunate to have one friend join me for walks three days of the week. Those three-mile walks continued throughout treatment. (I took off only a few days during chemo and four days after surgery.) We exercised our bodies and talked about the joys and trials of life. Those walks truly were therapeutic! So was the visualization I did. As we walked through the neighborhood passing rows and rows of houses, I would visualize squashing and destroying the bad cells and burying them. (I also used several helpful tapes, including *Positive Imagery for People with Cancer*, by Emmett E. Miller, M.D., and *Meditations for Enhancing Your Immune System*, by Bernie S. Siegel, M.D.)

I also found inspiration from the following poem, which was posted in the radiation oncology unit and now hangs in my living room:

WHAT CANCER CANNOT DO
Cancer is so limited . . .
It cannot cripple love, it cannot
Shatter hope,
It cannot corrode faith, it cannot
Destroy peace.
It cannot kill friendship, it cannot suppress memories,
It cannot silence courage, it cannot invade the soul,
It cannot steal eternal life,
It cannot conquer the spirit.

Author Unknown

One week after starting radiation, my friends helped me complete several 5+ mile hikes in the Columbia Gorge, where we viewed beautiful yellow wildflowers as the reward for our determination and perseverance. They encouraged me to take it one step at a time, just like the way I had to deal with the cancer treatments. One of my biggest achievements was climbing Mount St. Helens only two months after radiation (6 1/4 hours up and 4 hours down). I cried as we reached the top and my friend and I hugged each other and laughed. We asked someone to use our camera and take our picture as we raised our arms, beaming in triumph as the sunshine warmed our faces.

To celebrate my last day of radiation, my friends and I participated in the Relay for Life, a 24-hour fund-raiser for the American Cancer Society, which was held at a local track field. The track was lined with about 1,100 luminaries, white bags with lit candles, donated in memory or in honor of loved ones. Six candles were burning in my honor, thanks to the generosity of my family and friends. All of the survivors did the first lap, some walking, some running, and everyone else stood on the sidelines and clapped.

There's something about applause, especially when it comes from loving friends, that radiates a sense of joy and fills you with pride! There were 16 on our team that summer day. Just a few months later, a team of 12 of us participated in the Susan Komen Race for the Cure in Portland. It was awesome walking with 42,000 other women and men and seeing all the survivors wearing pink shirts. I felt so encouraged when I saw all the other women who had survived! It's also rewarding to know that money is being raised for breast cancer research that, hopefully, will continue to lead to more effective drugs and treatments with less adverse side effects.

When I started chemo, one of my daughter's friends sent me a symbolic survival kit, something I enjoyed so much that I've been making them for others and donating them to the local hospital oncology department, where nurses distribute them to new chemo patients. The card on the outside of the multicolored print, canvas bags tells you what's on the inside:

Survival Kit

A stick of gum to remind you to stick with it.

A candle to remind you to burn brightly.

A chocolate kiss to remind you that you are loved.

I'M LIVING PROOF that breast cancer is not the end of your life or activities—it just makes it more difficult and challenging. For me, every day is a blessing!

A match to light your fire when you feel burned out.

A Tootsie Roll to remind you not to bite off more than you can chew.

A pin to remind you to stay sharp.

Smarties to help you when you don't feel too smart.

A Starburst to give you a burst of energy on those days you don't have any.

A Lifesaver to help keep you afloat when you feel you are sinking.

A Snickers to remind you to take time to laugh.

A bag to help you keep it all together and to give you food for thought.

From the ♥ of a cancer survivor

In the future, I plan to continue making these survival kits and will donate my time to and participate in fund-raising races, as I live a life filled with many friends and a loving family. I am back to playing tennis two to three times a week and hiking, biking, walking, and cross-country skiing. I'm living proof that breast cancer is not the end of your life or activities—it just makes it more difficult and challenging. For me, every day is a blessing!

Justine McCollum, R.N.

Like a Rose in Your Garden

Y ou'll probably think I'm crazy when you read this, but breast cancer truly is the best thing that ever happened to me. If I were to write a book about it, I'd call it *The Joy of Breast Cancer*.

Why? Because breast cancer has helped me put things in perspective and understand what's important. It brought me closer to my husband and son, and it reunited me with my sister, from whom I'd been estranged for eight years.

From the day I was diagnosed at the age of 54, I felt as if luck had something to do with my cancer. It was in the middle of a typically hot, northern California summer when I awoke in the middle of the night to use the bathroom. As I made my way through the darkness, from my king-sized bed to the bathroom, my mind was so disoriented and my feet unsure, that I walked into a closed closet door and slammed my chest against its hard wooden surface.

The next day, I noticed that my right breast was bruised, and a week later, I saw that a lump had erupted underneath the bruise. My nurse's training taught me not to panic. "It's no big deal," I thought. "It's probably an accumulation of blood which leaked into the tissue spaces."

I also felt confident because three months earlier, I had a normal breast exam and mammography. I figured the internist I was scheduled to see in a week for my migraines could do a quick breast exam when I saw him. "It'll probably be a waste of his time," I told myself.

But it wasn't. He sent me to a surgeon, who ordered a needle biopsy. The results were much worse than I expected. "I'm sorry to tell you this," the surgeon said during a telephone call, "but the test results show that your lump is malignant."

I also heard him tell me that my breast cancer was the type that spread quickly and that it was in stage 2. Even though the news wasn't good, I was optimistic. "It's a good thing we scheduled that follow-up appointment, just in case, a week from now," I told the doctor.

After I hung up the phone, I walked out the back door into my one-acre yard. I could smell the fresh, sweet air and see the glory of my 170 rosebushes dressed in their magnificent colors of purple, apricot, and yellow and the trellis covered by climbing red roses. As I looked to the heavens, the sun warmed my face like it never had before. I almost became euphoric. I said to myself, "Oh, my God, this sun feels so good and I feel so healthy. I'm going to hang on to this moment as long as I can and for each day that follows!" That was the promise I made to myself, and I'd suggest you make it, too.

When I went back into the house, I felt great. Even though it was the fall season, I put on some Christmas music and I danced around the living room to a tune called "Good News." The song's words focused on Christ's birth and filled me with a sense of hope and joy and the celebration of life. I conjured up the blessings of Christmas as I freely danced and danced and danced, kicking my legs and waving my arms in circles to the music. "I'm not broken," I repeated to myself.

I was the first person in my family to be diagnosed with any form of cancer and knew it was important to let the others know of their possible risk. Even though my sister, Josie, and I hadn't talked in eight years because of a disagreement over my late mother's estate, I knew it was time to make up. It was right after Thanksgiving when I went into my bedroom, closed the door, and punched her number on the gray pads of my white telephone. When Josie heard my voice, she sounded surprised and happy. "I had to call you," I told her matter-of-factly. "I've been diagnosed with breast cancer."

The bad feelings quickly melted away on both sides of the phone as I told Josie, "Whatever has gone on in the past is over with, and what I'd like to do, if you're willing, is to start our life fresh from today and take it forward."

She agreed, and we talked after each of my doctor's appointments. My sister's married to a geneticist, and she wanted to know all the details so that she could do some research of her own. Josie and her husband also came from New Jersey to California to visit me about a month after I made that phone call. Their support, added to my husband's and children's love and caring, helped me feel stronger and more determined than ever to beat breast cancer!

It was important for me to respect my body for what it had to go through and to give it as much help, love, and support as I could.

I've heard people talk about *fighting* cancer and how some have gone into chemotherapy with an image of soldiers on horses firing rifles against the cancer cells. That made sense but it didn't work for me. I'm not a fighter. I'm a nurturer. I've always been employed in caring fields like nursing, social work, and teaching. So I decided that I was going to do what I knew best—nurture myself. It was important for me to respect my body for what it had to go through and to give it as much help, love, and support as I could. I had this vision of taking my body into my arms, cradling it, and rocking it like a baby. "There, there, you'll be all right," I cooed. "I'll help you through this, and we'll let the doctors and the medicine do the fighting."

The kindness of strangers helped, too. After I lost my hair from chemotherapy, I didn't wear a wig because it gave me a headache. The baseball cap didn't cover the fact that I was bald. I can't begin to tell you how many strangers came up to me and hugged me, smiled at me, and said, "I'll pray for you."

Grocery store clerks, the folks at the cleaners, and the man at the nursery asked how I was doing. The nursery man, however, floored me with his special gift. "You are like a rose in your garden," the normally quiet man said. "You may have a black spot or mold or fungus, but you stand tall and you hold your head high and you show your beautiful colors."

His kind words took away my fear of being in public. After that encounter, I walked through a crowd making eye contact and people smiled back at me. Their faces spoke volumes.

During my chemotherapy, I watched a video of Riverdance, a fast-stepping, high-powered Irish dance troupe. I couldn't move, but at least I could watch the dancers furiously tap dancing on the stage. I envisioned myself jumping in the air, just like them.

Dancing, I closed my eyes and I imagined myself going through the motions. It helped me feel centered and grounded.

I joined dance movement therapy classes for breast cancer survivors. It was through these classes that I was lifted out of my depression because, through my body of movement and dance, I was able to express my emotions when the words wouldn't come and get in touch with what I was going through —it made me whole again. I got back my identity, felt centered and grounded, and was Justine again, not just a cancer patient. One day after a class, I returned home and was working at my desk. I opened an overhead cabinet and out flew a small piece of paper. It was a receipt from my expired nursing license. I saw it as a special message and called the telephone number on the receipt. I had 30 days to renew my license or I'd have to take the nursing boards all over again.

After I renewed my license, I went back into nursing, loving it more than ever. I'm trying to make some good changes, too. I'm working on getting a VCR, a monitor, and breast self-exam videos in all Kaiser Medical radiology department waiting rooms.

I also happily talk with women who are referred to me through the grapevine about their breast cancer fears and questions. I'm very blessed to be able to provide both medical knowledge and emotional support. Many of these women tell me I'm their guardian angel. I don't know about that, but I do believe that things happen for a reason. Even though my parents were atheists and taught me not to believe in God, I do. That faith gives me a sense of peace and hope, and it feels good inside. I know that the sunshine on my face the day I went into my backyard after hearing my diagnosis was God-given. Just like the many glorious years I've lived beyond that time. I don't want to be just a breast cancer survivor. I always want to be a breast cancer thriver.

Joan Halperin

Jumping the Waves

I t was spring 1979 when I went in to see Lennie Gutner, my internist and friend, for an annual checkup. I felt wonderful. I'd finally bounced back from the exhaustion and depression over my mother's death from uterine cancer in 1976. My kids were thriving. Our daughter was in college, loving it, and had a boyfriend, Lloyd, whom she was wild about. Our son was getting some acclaim as a blues guitarist. And I had a job as a therapeutic nursery schoolteacher at a clinic near our home. I'd thought up a program where I had mothers of young children in my group teach each other skills while the children were in class. One mother taught knitting, another cooking, another taught how to write letters applying for benefits. And I felt proud. Also, the empty nest syndrome didn't disturb me. We lived in a suburb near New York City. My husband and I went to the opera, concerts, and theater. I was full of energy, ready to work and to run into the city at a moment's notice.

After Lennie examined me, he said, "Let's go talk in my office." Since this was part of our regular routine, I wasn't the least bit concerned. However, when Lennie sat down, he looked worried.

"Look, Joanie," he said. "I feel a tiny lump, perhaps the size of a pea, in your right breast. I don't think a mammogram would pick it up at this point. If I were you, I'd wait a few weeks. Chances are it will surface and blend into the granular tissue in your breast until it grows a bit and becomes more defined. But I can tell you, it doesn't have the feel of a malignancy. It rolls around your chest. That's a good sign."

I've never been a patient person and waiting isn't in my vocabulary, so as soon as I was out of Lennie's office, I rushed to the nearest pay phone and called my husband.

"Lennie felt a lump," I whispered, not wanting anyone to hear. My mouth was dry. I kept tapping my feet. Time to get moving and find out if I was going to follow in my mother's footsteps. I could see her wild eyes, her bald head, just before she died from uterine cancer. "I'm going to schedule a mammogram right this minute," I said. My husband tried to reassure me that everything would be okay, but I detected worry in his voice.

I went to a radiologist the next day. She sandwiched my right breast in the X-ray machine. As I lay on a paper-covered examining table, a light cotton gown wrapped around my upper body, I waited for the results. "Please, God," I prayed as I looked at the ceiling, "don't let it be cancer."

When a doctor came in, he had a smile on his face and shook my hand. "Congratulations. We saw nothing," he said. But since Dr. Gutner felt a lump, I would have another examination in a few weeks.

I couldn't stand the thought of waiting and was relieved when my husband told me he had been able to schedule an appointment with a top surgeon the following week.

As I drove to the surgeon's office, I kept lifting up my navy blue sweater as I drove, digging for the lump with my fingers. One moment it was there, a small round pea, hard and definite. The next, it had disappeared. I kept examining myself until I pulled into the parking garage.

When I checked in at the desk, the nurse handed me a long questionnaire. My hand was shaking. Why couldn't someone else fill this out? As I looked up from my paperwork, I noticed an older couple huddled together on the chintz sofa. She wore a shapeless navy blue dress. Had she had a breast removed? I stared into space until a nurse called my name.

"Just take everything off except your underpants. And here's a paper robe. Back part open," the nurse ordered. (I never understood why the back part was supposed to be left open when it's the front part they were going to examine.)

"He's extremely busy today. So wait on the edge of the table so you can lay down the minute he comes in," she said before quickly leaving the room.

"I'm not a 'thing'," I wanted to snap. "Why can't he wait for me to lie down?" No one was there to listen.

When the surgeon came into the examining room, I noticed that everything about him seemed sterile: his silver hair, his white jacket, the perfectly clean hands and trimmed fingernails. "I have your doctor's report and the mammogram shows that everything is clear. Lie down please."

As I lay, breasts exposed, on the paper-lined stainless steel examining table, the surgeon used both hands to search for the lump. His fingers roamed up, down, and around, pressing and turning the skin as he tried to locate the pea-sized invader. But somehow, miraculously, it had disappeared. Was Lennie wrong? Had he imagined something that wasn't there? I was jubilant.

"What makes you think there's a lump?" the surgeon asked. He sounded irritated, as if I had been wasting his time.

I mumbled something about my doctor feeling it, as the surgeon left the room.

When I called my husband with the good news that I was cancer free and didn't need to be checked again, he wasn't as jubilant as I.

"That sounds strange," he said. "Why don't you call the nurse at the office and ask to be examined again?"

Even though I thought Stan was being a worrywart, I followed his advice and made the call. The nurse found my chart and read it to me—the surgeon wanted me to come back in six weeks. "I wondered why you rushed out of the office," she said. "I was going to call you later this afternoon."

The second examination was all business as I followed the surgeon's cold instructions to hold my arms up behind my head. I remember there were magnificent black-and-white photos of the Greek islands on the examining room wall. I studied the photos as his hands explored my breasts once more. I felt his fingers reexamine the spot Lennie had found. He went over and over that area of my right breast. "There's a small lump. I'm going to aspirate it if I can. If we can get fluid out, you won't need to go to the hospital."

I kept thinking, "I want my mother."

As the surgeon pushed the needle into my breast, he commented, "I'm afraid it's too small to aspirate. But it rolls around. Good sign. I recommend that I biopsy it at Mount Sinai Hospital next week just to make sure we don't miss a malignancy. So please set up an appointment at the desk. If you have questions, ask my head nurse."

I was 50 years old. I had spent years fighting against depression. Now just when I had turned the corner and was feeling more upbeat, my life was being threatened. Those seven days of waiting for the biopsy were torture. I experienced terror when I awoke in the mornings, when I bathed, and when I went to the movies.

The surgeon asked me to sign a consent form when I arrived at the hospital. I refused because I didn't want a blanket consent to permit a surgeon to perform a mastectomy if he found cancer. I'd just read Rose Kushner's book entitled *Why Me?: What Every Woman Should Know About Breast Cancer to Save Her Life,* in which women had been warned not to allow surgeons to make medical decisions without first obtaining the patient's consent.

"I really want to decide with you, what I do next, if I have cancer," I informed the surgeon, finally saying the C word out loud.

The surgeon muttered something about women libbers. But he crossed out the section giving blanket approval. "See you in the morning," he said and stalked out of the room.

I was informed of the results when I was in the recovery room: a malignant tumor in a milk duct. I remember being very cold. I kept asking for blankets. But I was hot inside. "F*** you! F*** you!" I cursed the surgeon. "You told me it looked benign." Ignoring my verbal venom, the surgeon said he wanted to perform a modified mastectomy in two weeks.

Refusing to give up the one-sided fight, I responded, "I'm losing a breast. How is that moderate?"

The day Dr. L took off the bandages, I quickly slipped an old white Shetland sweater over my mutilated self. But that night, Stan insisted we look at me together. We stood side by side in front of a floor-length mirror. At first I kept my eyes shut, and when I slowly opened them, I saw the reflection of a woman who was half boy on one side and the sexy me on the other. The surgeon hadn't just chopped off my breast, but half my life. Stan pulled me toward him, away from the dreaded mirror, and we both began to cry. I wept without restraint. I would never be the same again. Never.

"You're beautiful," he said and kissed my left breast and then the flat side of me. A thin red scar divided me in half.

We hugged. "Not too hard," I warned. "The bad side is sore."

"There's no bad side. You know you look more like who you are," he quipped. "A bit quirky and lopsided. That's the girl I fell in love with. An offbeat kid."

We'd been married 27 years. Some of it had been rough going. He was practical. I was a dreamer. He tended to want to hunker down at home. I was an adventurer. I was the kite. He was the string. Now we both needed each other more than ever. He needed to know I would fly again. And I had never been more in need of stability. We talked about our lives, started making plans.

"We're going to take a winter vacation this year," he said. No more saving every penny for a rainy day. I brought home some Club Med brochures. We stretched out on the bed and studied the pictures of grinning Caribbean vacationers who were snorkeling and sipping piña coladas.

My friends planned excursions, invited me to the movies, for lunch dates, to concerts. I was difficult, testy, demanding. Sure, it was easy for them to treat me well—they had normal bodies! I was now a freak.

Then something happened that began to turn the tide. When I returned to my job as head teacher at the clinic, I found that my assistant teacher, who'd taken over my responsibilities when I was sick, had no intention of relinquishing her authority. Colleagues informed me that she was eager to permanently acquire my job. That old fight in me was activated. There's no way I'm leaving the job I love—she's not going to have a chance to even get near it, I promised myself. I informed her that I was feeling great and that I'd be back, better than ever!

The mother's knitting group had crocheted a king-sized afghan for me. I lifted it up in the air, admiring the rows of greens, violets, and blues—my favorite colors.

Another turning point was when we went to Martha's Vineyard, where we had a summer home. Our crowd had started nude bathing a few years before. We were late bloomers! In our 50s, some of us were lumpy and big hipped. In the water, we felt smooth and light and we relished the freedom of being naked.

The first week of vacation, we went to Gay Head Beach. My women friends, Gloria, Helen, and Alice, kept complimenting me on my new bathing suits. I hated the high necklines that hid my concave chest, the pocket hidden inside that held the prosthesis, the muted blues and discreet black colors. I sensed their unease. As the women began to undress and the men shed their suits, I felt I couldn't bear it. Every woman had two breasts. How could I tolerate anyone but Stan seeing my body? Judy, my 19-year-old daughter, sat next to me reading a book. She looked up at me, gave me a thumbs-up sign.

I needed to be alone, so I walked down the beach by myself, filled with self-pity. What I didn't know was that Judy was following me, and she saw me standing at the edge of the shore, my body shaking as I cried.

"Take off your suit, Mom. I brought us both towels," my daughter urged me from behind.

"Suppose a child sees me?"

"Then that child will see a brave woman. Come on," she started to poke at me. "Off with the suit!"

We stood at the shoreline and stripped. The blue flowered mastectomy suit hit the sand. Within its cup rested the silicone prosthesis. I crossed my arms around my chest. I felt the sea breeze, heard the waves, welcomed the touch of Judy's arm linked into mine. I began to feel as if my mind and my body were one again. I reclaimed ownership of my body, something I had refused to do since the mastectomy. As I let my arms drop to my sides, I heard Judy yell, "The last one in is a wimp!"

We raced into those cool waters, screaming with glee as the water enveloped our bodies. When I took those first strokes, I felt the old sense of freedom and zest returning into my soul. Water covered me, jostled me, rippled through my legs, my breast, my flat side, crashed above my head. Judy and I began jumping the waves.

I started belting out a nursery school song that I often sang with my class. "The eensy teensy spider went up the waterspout. Down came the rain and washed the spider out."

Judy joined in. "Out came the sun and dried up all the rain. And the eensy teensy spider went up the spout again."

We began howling that song into the waves.

I could see the shore, the great red cliffs, the tiny sea

Come to think about it, aren't we all required to jump the waves if we're going to get past our personal demons?

terns, and the stands of seaweed. I had a wonderful husband. Great kids. I'd kept my job. I felt myself shedding the anger. That anger had been necessary. It had kick-started me into life again. I was a lopsided, funny woman. I had gifts to give. And over the last months, I'd received more love than I knew I had coming to me. My daughter had instinctively known it was time for me to face my fears. By stripping, I'd faced the risk of exposure. I was preparing for the years ahead. Because, come to think about it, aren't we all required to jump the waves if we're going to get past our personal demons? I was going to get knocked down time after time. But right then, in that cool healing water, I knew it was worth the struggle.

"You better not pull that one on me again." I tipped my head at the omnipotent one in the sky. "Enough is enough." And I thought about my son a moment. He'd decided not to go to college because he loved playing the guitar. He'd jumped the waves, too. And I remembered him praising me for my decision not to sign a blanket consent form. "Hey, Mom, that took guts. Standing up to the establishment," he'd said.

Emerging from the water, Judy and I draped the towels around our shivering bodies. I slipped my suit on. And we walked victoriously, arm in arm, back toward our friends.

Stan waved toward us as we approached. "You're back," he said.

"I do believe I am!" I said, wrapping my arm around him as I flopped onto a beach chair and looked triumphantly at the rolling waves in front of us.

Lori Misicka

Diagnosis: Canceritis

It was just a little bump. A very little red mosquito-bite-looking bump. It was on my stomach, slightly above and just to the left of my belly button, and I noticed it one day while I was taking a shower.

"Hmmm," I thought, "that's a weird place for a skin tag." I have many assorted skin tags, moles, beauty marks, age spots, and other skin decorations too insignificant to even have names, but I'd never had one on my stomach. I didn't bother thinking about it again.

Until the next day. Once again in the shower, I casually noted that the little red bump was still there, but then I promptly forgot about it as soon as I turned off the water.

On day three, when I saw the bump had not gone away, I started getting nervous. I couldn't remember ever having had a red skin tag before, and, of course, there was the fact that it was on my stomach, which had never happened before either. I found myself surreptitiously lifting my shirt every couple of hours throughout the next couple of days to check the status of the bump, and every time, I saw that it was still there and became more alarmed.

Of course, I tried to talk myself down. "Think rationally," I told myself. "Try to stay in the present moment," I advised. "Remain calm," I pleaded. But every time my fingers strayed over the area and felt that slightly raised spot, my heart skipped a beat and my breath caught.

I lived in a steadily increasing state of panic for one week—seven very long days—the arbitrary amount of time I've always given any physical weirdness to run its course before taking it seriously. Over the years, there had actually been times when I couldn't remember the exact day I'd first noticed a certain ache or spot; that was not the case this time. This time, I remembered the exact moment I first noticed the little red bump, and every day that passed with it still being there on my stomach was one day closer to the day I'd have to acknowledge it as something to be addressed. And I definitely did not want it to be something that had to be addressed. Even so, it was all I could do to make myself wait those seven days. Living with that little red bump on my stomach was one of the hardest things I've ever had to do, and as soon as the seventh day arrived, I did what any woman who has just finished breast cancer treatment would do: I ran to my doctor's office as fast as I could!

Breast cancer is an interesting animal. Even though I knew that there were many breast cancer survivors out there walking around living their lives, when I was diagnosed I immediately thought I was going to die. And pretty much right away. But as the days and the weeks and the months went by, I came to realize that I just might be one of the lucky ones who made it, and so I began to relax a little.

As strange as that sounds, it's true. By that time, I was fully involved in my treatment plan and I was on a mission, doing everything I could to become healthy again. I tried to cover all the bases: combining conventional medicine—chemo, surgery, and radiation—with other not-so-conventional forms of treatment, like prayer, meditation, and visualization. Waiting in my oncologist's office one day, I saw a flyer about a dance movement therapy class exclusively for breast cancer patients and survivors, and I signed up for it. After the 12-week class ended,

As the days and the weeks and the months went by, I came to realize that I just might be one of the lucky ones who made it.

some of us got together and formed our own group, and we met monthly to continue our healing activities in art and music and movement. I also joined a weekly face-to-face support group. I became an expert in my kind of breast cancer and in all the standard and experimental treatments for it by raiding every bookstore in town. I learned to use e-mail and participated daily in an e-mail support group specifically for people with inflammatory breast cancer, the type I'd been diagnosed with. I began surfing the Net, and I drove my oncologist crazy with all my questions about strange and bizarre therapies I'd read about on dubious Web sites. I'd bring her information about coffee and apricot pit enemas or shark cartilage or essiac tea or high doses of vitamin C or the latest study on one of her treatment recommendations, and she'd greet me either with a lively discussion of medical issues or with an exasperated shake of her head over my need to explore every option.

In other words, I started to feel like I had a handle on this cancer thing. I felt like I had some control.

And then, after nine months of total immersion in medical appointments, procedures, and theories with 100 percent of my focus directed to my healing, I finished treatment.

Wow! I was ecstatic and relieved and grateful and even a bit proud that I had survived all the poking and prodding and probing and plotting. "Now," I thought, "my life can get back to normal."

The euphoria of surviving and finishing treatment lasted about a week. All of a sudden, my days were empty—no more radiation treatments messing up my daily schedule, no doctor appointments, no tests, no researching the next step in the treatment plan. It hit me that I was no longer doing anything to fend off the cancer, that I wasn't doing anything to prevent it from coming back. I felt like a tightrope walker performing without a net. I no longer had any control.

So I became obsessed with checking my body for signs that "it" was back, not that I really had any idea of what those signs might be. I looked for lumps and bumps all over my body. Cysts that had been in residence for decades became suspect. Moles that had been part of my physical landscape from birth were examined daily for changes. I didn't stop at a breast self-exam; I performed total body exams. Every shower became an agonizing torturous event as I checked and double-checked every inch of my body for evidence that "it" had taken over again. I had a full-blown, hard-core case of canceritis.

Yes, canceritis—the most common and least treatable long-term side effect of breast cancer. You see, the body is remarkable in its healing abilities, but the mind is another matter altogether.

The first time I encountered the canceritis phenomenon was a few months after I was diagnosed. I was on the phone with my mother, a 45-year survivor, and she was telling me how great her surgeon had been all those years ago when she'd gone through her breast cancer experience. She especially appreciated his sense of humor, and she laughed as she recalled one visit when, after listing for him all her aches and pains that proved the cancer had returned, he asked her very seriously where she'd received her medical degree. When my mother told me this story, I remember rolling my eyes and thinking how incredibly paranoid she was.

So a few months later, here I was doing the very same thing over a little red bump! I didn't feel too bad about it, though, because by that time I'd met and spoken to many women going through their own breast cancer experiences, and every one of them had canceritis to some degree. Some called their doctors almost daily with symptoms, some just thought about calling their doctors with symptoms, but all of them were almost preternaturally aware of every nuance of their bodies. And for most of them, the symptoms had begun shortly after their treatment had ended.

Hair grows back, nausea goes away, blood cell counts return to normal—the body heals. But the mind seems to gnaw on that cancer thing like a dog gnaws on a bone: compulsively for a time and then burying it and then digging it up to gnaw on it again and then burying it and then digging it up again and on and on. There are lots of different medications and therapies to heal the body's wounds, but there seems to be only one treatment for the mind. An understanding doctor helps, and so does the ability to remain calm and not panic. But the magic bullet for alleviating the symptoms of canceritis is time. And the more time that passes, the less canceritis you have.

Now that she's 45 years out, when my mother gets a cough, her first thought is not, "Oh, my God, I have lung cancer." When her elbow hurts, she doesn't immediately think, "I must call the doctor, it's elbow cancer." After all the years and colds and flus and sore throats and various and sundry ailments, the possibility that the cancer's come back is pretty far down the list of what it could be. Instead, for my mother, a cough's a cough, a sore elbow's a sore elbow. Nothing more, nothing less. Forty-five years of time has, for all intents and purposes, cured my mother of canceritis.

However, it had been only about 45 days for me when I discovered that little red bump on my stomach, and so the possibility that the cancer had come back was pretty much number one on my list of what it could be. Hence, my race to the doctor.

The doctor said that it was probably nothing. I asked how she knew it was nothing. She said that it didn't look like cancer, didn't feel like cancer, wasn't in a logical place for cancer to be. I repeated my question. She then explained to me that just because I've had cancer doesn't mean I'm not a candidate for other more benign illnesses and conditions. (Hardly fair, as far as I'm concerned. It seems to me that I've more than filled my quota for health issues!) And I said that sounded reasonable to me, but how did she know it was nothing?

Just to get rid of me, I think, she sent me to the dermatologist, who told me it was probably nothing. I asked how she knew it was nothing. She said that it didn't look like cancer, didn't feel like cancer, wasn't in a logical place for cancer to be. I repeated my question. Just to get rid of me, I think, she removed that little red bump, did a biopsy of it, and proved that it was indeed nothing.

I felt a lot better without that little red bump on my stomach (of course, now there's a little red scar instead), but I realized how foolish I'd been. It's certainly understandable that I would immediately suspect cancer and it was even responsible of me to consult a doctor, but I really did go a little crazy about it, insisting on a second opinion and not resting until a biopsy had been done. That canceritis definitely had me going.

So I decided to take a lesson from my mother and think twice before diagnosing myself with cancer every time I have a little ache or a little red bump. And I also decided to stop the anatomical examinations in the shower every day. I mean, I know there are no guarantees, but why go looking for trouble? Why live the rest of your life worrying about every little something that pops up?

And I plan on making those changes just as soon as I get back from the doctor. You see, I've got this pain in my finger and . . .

From Russia with Love

When Stephen, my husband of three years, and I decided it was time to have children, it wasn't as easy for me to get pregnant as we had hoped. My doctor suggested that having surgery would increase my chances of conceiving.

The surgeon thought it would be a good time to also get a biopsy of the tissue in my right breast because of some densities that were felt during earlier exams. "It's just a precaution," he said.

I was more worried about the chances of the surgery's success to increase conception rather than whether the biopsy would reveal that I had breast cancer. After all, it was just a precaution, as the surgeon said, and I wasn't considered a high risk. I was going to be under the influence of anesthesia anyway. What did I have to lose?

Unfortunately, the biopsy revealed that I did have breast cancer. "The good news," my surgeon said, "is that your chances of survival are between 80 and 90 percent."

Stephen and I didn't feel like that was something to celebrate. I had just lost a 10 to 20 percent chance to live. And what about having children? How could I think about creating a life when I was worried about losing my own?

"We can always adopt," I reassured Stephen when we learned that my chances of ever getting pregnant were destroyed by the chemotherapy following a mastectomy. I had considered the possibility of adopting as a single parent before I got married. I knew that in spite of having cancer my desire to have children had not waned. But I was worried about my chances of being able to adopt. Would a person with a history of breast cancer be able to pass inspection by the rulers of the adoption kingdom?

Before trying to adopt, we decided to wait five years. Our hope was that being five years free of cancer, I would look cured to the home study people and to the Russian authorities to whom we had turned to adopt children. We knew it was a gamble, but it was one we were willing to take.

We had decided that Russia was the best place for us to find our daughters because we would not run the risk of losing them over a nasty custody battle like the ones we had read about in the newspapers in the United States.

> *If there's one thing that cancer teaches you, it's that you don't have time to waste.*

If there's one thing that cancer teaches you, it's that you don't have time to waste. We wanted to adopt older children, two girls about five to eight years of age, because we were too old for babies and figured they needed us as much as we needed them. We were both getting older and thought that if,

God forbid, either of us died early, the girls would have each other. We also had backup plans for relatives to raise the girls, if need be. (We weren't trying to be maudlin, just practical.)

We had to travel to Russia to pick up Alicia and Jessica, two five-year-old girls who were about to become the daughters for whom we yearned. How do you fall in love with two little, complete strangers who don't even speak your language? How could we not? We were able to see Jessica on a video the Russian government sent to us. Her dark blond hair was short. She had beautiful blue eyes and she wore a pink dress. Jessica was just beautiful!

As we boarded the plane to go to Russia, I thought, "Phooey on you, cancer! Not only am I alive, but I'm going to become a mother! We are finally going to have and to become a family!"

At the orphanage, we first met Jessica when she came into the director's office. She would recognize us, we knew, because months ahead of time, we had sent her a photo album of us, our home, our dog, and our two cats. We had information about us translated into Russian. When she walked into the room, Jessica stood at the door, looked at us, and asked, "Mama? Papa?" and jumped into my lap.

As I hugged her and cried, all I could think was, "How little and beautiful you are!"

It was absolutely the perfect start to our family, and there was no hesitation for any of us.

Next we met Alicia, who did not know that we were going to have her join our family. A facilitator had told us about her when we were in Russia, and when we met this beautiful five-and-a-half-year-old with short medium-brown hair and bluish green eyes, we held our breath as she examined the photo album we had sent to Jessica. After a few moments, Alicia looked up at us and asked, "Mama? Papa?" There wasn't a dry eye in the room!

Many people have told us that we were brave to have adopted the girls. I don't know about that. The way I see it is that no one knows how long she has to live, breast cancer or not. From where I'm standing, I see a bright future with two daughters who never would have entered my heart if it weren't for my diagnosis. We did not ignore breast cancer. We just worked around it.

The Patient

One week after my 35th birthday, I was diagnosed with breast cancer. By accident, I had found a tiny lump on my right breast when I was applying sunscreen, which was ironic because I hardly ever used the stuff.

Both of my doctors thought the lump was benign because they said it wasn't the hard consistency of a malignant tumor.

"Wait three months," they advised.

Not wanting to wait at all to see if the tumor was going to change in size or not, I responded with the best question I ever posed: "What would you do if I were your wife?"

Their answer was different then. In a matter of days, they did a biopsy and breast cancer was confirmed.

I had two young children at the time. Kelly was three and Cody was five, and I was so busy with them and trying to stay healthy that feeling sorry for myself was never an option. (I was probably sadder about my son going off to kindergarten than I was about my cancer.) I'm not going to lie and tell you I didn't cry about the diagnosis. Of course I did. Cancer gave me a quick glimpse of the possibility of not being able to watch my kids grow up and not being there for them. Let me tell you, that possibility made me so determined to do whatever it took to increase my chances of survival that I welcomed the difficult surgeries and chemotherapy, because I knew they were being done to help me survive.

In less than a year, I had eight surgeries, including a double mastectomy. None of that kept me from teaching aerobics and doing personal training. I taught 12 classes a week during my chemotherapy treatments. (Yes, I'm crazy!) I believe that all of the exercise and teaching, coupled with my positive attitude, helped me not only to survive cancer but to come out of it as a better person. Teaching aerobics throughout chemotherapy made me tougher, and that made me a better fighter. I proved to myself and others that breast cancer could not stop the fulfilling life I had.

My friends and the students in my YMCA classes in Austin, Texas, buoyed my spirits with phone calls and delivered dinners, not to mention a maid for six months.

I did take a month off from teaching to heal from my double mastectomy, but as I had promised my students, I was back just one day short of a month from the surgery. I'm not a superwoman, but I do believe that being in shape helped me heal quickly and motivated me to keep my promise to return within weeks. When I returned I didn't overdo it because some members of my senior aerobics class watched over me like mother hens. When it looked like I was doing too much, Leslie would say, "Amy, you can rest. We know what to do." Or Annell would tell me, "Put down the heavy weights. You need to be healing, not building muscle." Two of the seniors had experienced breast cancer and were so understanding of what I was enduring.

It's been two years since my surgery, and so far I've trained five breast cancer survivors. When survivors find out that I'm one, too, it excites them about starting a workout program and they're comforted to know that "one of their own" is doing the training. I can adjust the weight lifting because we've all had the axillary node surgery. When these survivors feel better and have more energy from exercising, I feel so rewarded! I've noticed for myself and others that when you feel fit, you feel better overall and your attitude certainly improves. (My surgeon believes that attitude is about 90 percent of the prognosis.)

> *I'VE NOTICED FOR myself and others that when you feel fit, you feel better overall and your attitude certainly improves.*

My attitude turned playful when I had reconstruction immediately after my mastectomy. During a follow-up with my plastic surgeon, I asked about tattoos on my breast. "What about hearts, sort of like my badge of courage?" I asked.

"I've waited years to have someone do something crazy!" she said, hugging me.

The way I see it is, hey, I'm just glad to be here and why not do something fun?

I had the best doctors and surgeons and I felt honored when my oncologist asked me to be his "poster child." He and his staff were designing a brochure for new patients, and they wanted me to be on the front of it. There I am in a black-and-white photo, waist up, wearing a black sleeveless knit shirt, with the words "The Patient" above my head. And over my chest is a description about my diagnosis, my surgeries, and how exercise has helped me stay in shape and how I have helped others.

I hope to continue inspiring others through exercise that includes running triathlons, the first of which I ran four months after finishing chemotherapy. I joined Team Survivor, a national nonprofit organization for women with breast cancer, whose goal is to encourage survivors to get into and keep physically fit through exercise.

If you would have told me five years ago that I would be racing in triathlons and loving it, I would have laughed. But after what I've been through, it's just an honor to be able to compete. No matter what my time is in the races, I know that I am already a winner.

Fifty-Five and Alive!

There are months you remember and months you forget. Most of life's months merge, blend, and are largely forgotten. September 2001 will always be my month to remember. On September 11, the World Trade Center twin towers went down. On September 25, my routine mammogram indicated a suspicious mass, followed shortly by The Diagnosis. Both events have striking parallels: terrorist cells and cancer cells—unseen deadly forces at work night and day to bring me down, swept along by uncontrollable events, fear, anger, frustration, sorrow, and grief. I was under attack from without and within. There was no safe haven, no place to hide, and few thoughts that weren't consumed by potential disaster. I rationed my tears between my family and the families touched by our national tragedy. In the ensuing weeks, we gathered facts, America and I. Who are the culprits? How and when to retaliate? We both settled on strategic strikes against an unseen enemy lurking in the caves beneath an austere landscape. We were at war with forces diametrically opposed. My cancer, their Taliban. Both were on a mission, and coexistence seemed impossible. You don't negotiate with cancer or extremists.

By the time the anthrax threat kicked in, life had become totally surreal. I am an "in control" woman, and my world was definitely out of control. The road I thought I was traveling suddenly dropped off the edge. There were no signposts, no maps, no certain destination. For the first time in my life, I could not see my future. All bets were off. As world governments sought to spin events with patriotic fervor, I went to work on the only things I felt I could control—attitude and behavior. "They can get to my body," I said, "but not my spirit. It's mine, I own it, and I won't give it up." Our country won't either. As long as there is breath left in me and in America, we will prevail.

Usually closemouthed about my personal troubles, I decided to take a different tack this time. I knew I could not get through this alone. I had to share the emotional burden with others in the hope that the weight of it would be diminished if my friends helped with the load. So I told everyone who would listen that I had breast cancer. It is not easy to deliver such news to people who care about you, but I did it, and I also asked for help, something I usually reserve as a last resort. I asked people who pray to pray for me. I asked people who do not worship to send me positive thoughts. I asked everyone for their most outrageous jokes. It worked. I found great comfort in accepting humor as therapy and dispensing it myself as a tonic for those I had inadvertently caused pain. Referring to the radiology room as "my personal tanning salon" changed the nature of my experience for friends and family. For me, humor had the ability of taking the horror out of the horrible.

By being forthright about my diagnosis, I found others living with breast cancer and drained them of their sage advice. It seems that everyone knows someone who has had breast cancer. I talked with friends who then put me in touch with other friends. Surprisingly, I also discovered acquaintances who, unbeknownst to me, were breast cancer survivors. Many had gone through much worse than I had to face, and their experiences provided a map to follow. Through them I found

> *It seems that everyone knows someone who has had breast cancer.*

firsthand descriptions of what it is like to be on the front line of cancer treatment. They provided the color commentary. Through them I saw what my future might hold. Most important, through them I came to the realization that if they could endure it, I knew I could as well. Nothing soothes fears like the sight and sound of a survivor.

I discovered that people in my life cared for me more than I knew. I might have lived my entire life without realizing the power of such declarative caring. Friends from New York, Florida, Colorado, and Kansas decided it was time for a visit. I saw more long-distance friends in the six months following surgery than I had in years. My work colleagues and neighbors provided a daily source of positive thought and caring. At night when it was tough to sleep, I'd wrap myself in those prayers and good wishes, as I would bundle against the winter wind. I'd drift off to sleep, warm, secure, and protected.

I also felt a sense of gratitude. My cancer was caught early before it spread to the nodes (not to say that the microcritters hadn't gotten out some other way, but statistically the prognosis was good). All other biological markers were favorable. I had medical coverage. I wasn't an Afghan refugee sitting beneath a hot burka, undiagnosed, on the border with Pakistan. What if English wasn't my first language, what if I had zero ability to grapple with the medical concepts, what if I had no medical coverage, what if I were stationed at the North Pole and had to do my own surgery and chemotherapy?

I had a lumpectomy with sentinel node biopsy the day after my 55th birthday. I've had dry cleaning take longer. In by six, out by eleven. No lunch served, not even a bag of airplane peanuts for a snack. Like a half-day kindergartner, I was given some juice and sent home for a nap. Three days later, I was back to work and resumed my thrice-weekly aerobics class. I had little pain or even discomfort. There was a dent in my breast, but it was more whole than not. I was still alive.

Radiation became as routine as stopping for groceries on the way home from work. Star Wars-type technology has made it possible to pinpoint radiation trajectories with astounding accuracy—or so I'm told. So I'm a little tired. So what, if it would extend my life? I have faith that the machines, the technicians, the radiologist, the oncologist, the studies, the statistics, the pills, the whole works will pull me through this. My life depends on the skills of strangers. Trust comes first and, ultimately, faith kicks in.

At the end of the week of my surgery, I hosted a potluck supper at my house for 18 friends (I had, after all, been home for three days and had had time to clean). Everyone brought wonderful food and drink, including my boss's offering of two bottles of champagne. Toward the end of the evening, we "toasted the tumor." Gathered on our deck overlooking Austin's Lake Travis with upraised glasses, in unison, my friends offered their wishes for a good, long life. "To Liz" drifted out over the lake and quelled the surrounding darkness, internal and external. It just doesn't get any better than that.

Breast cancer has reminded me that I am going to die, maybe sooner than I thought. But death can't be all that difficult; people do it all the time. I am on good terms with the concept and prospect. It holds no overly negative connotations, except the sadness of leaving my friends and family behind, especially my husband, whose coping skills are minimal and for whom life would be difficult without me. Death is a transition—for believers, a transition to a better place, not so much a separation as the ultimate unification. And yet I am determined to go the distance in this life. They'll have to take me kicking and screaming all the way to the goal line. In a journal I was given as a cancer patient freebie, one of the chapter headings was "Am I Going to Die?" I burst out laughing and said to the book, as if it could hear, "Don't be silly. Of course I am going to die." I just don't know when, where, or by what means. Even with cancer, I can still get run over crossing the street on any given Monday through Sunday.

When I was a junior in high school, my father went to work one morning and never returned, because he dropped dead of a heart attack. His untimely and tragic death made me wonder about the changes he might have made in the way he lived his life if he had had some warning. What unfinished business did he leave behind, things left undone or unsaid?

In comparison, I'm glad to have a little heads-up. The wonderful thing about remembering that I am going to die is that it reminds me to make the most of being alive.

I have become more spirit than body. There is a newfound detachment. I have accepted the things I cannot change and have gone about the business of changing and safeguarding my attitude, which I can control. Fearfulness, fed by uncertainty, has turned to defiance; bewilderment has morphed into an understanding that, no matter what, I'll be okay and those I love will be okay. I hate ambiguity and lack patience. Breast cancer delivers both in crate-size containers. Waiting for lab results alone tests one's ability to remain calm and concentrate on the tasks at hand. Detail-oriented and prone to worrying about trifles, I now have a "cancer measuring stick" that reduces mountains to molehills. As the saying goes, "Don't sweat the small stuff and everything is small stuff." I now thoroughly understand that the ebb and flow of daily challenges are of little consequence when stacked up against my own mortality. I no longer waste a lot of time and energy on things that simply don't matter in the long run. I still show up on time. I still wash the clothes—I meet all previously performed obligations. But the perfectionist in me has become a couch potato. Sunrises and sunsets are significant, as are the exquisite quality of the morning air, the way wildflowers pop up after a rain, a genuine smile, an embrace from a friend, a husband's gift of weekend flowers. Time is precious and elongated. I realized that an awful lot of life can be just plain silly or wasted. But no more.

My brother always said that you never get 100 percent from life, that somewhere in the 80th percentile was more realistic. Ironically, my five-year survival rate is around about 87 percent—pretty good by my brother's standard. Ultimately, it is all about maximizing what you are given to work

> *Sunrises and sunsets are significant, as are the exquisite quality of the morning air, the way wildflowers pop up after a rain, a genuine smile, an embrace from a friend, a husband's gift of weekend flowers.*

with. Some folks can work wonders with just a few talents. Others squander everything they've got. Cancer has taken something from me, but it has also added new things. Important things like the quality of friendship and life itself. I will celebrate all that I have been given for as long as I live.

The future? Who knows? Be it bombing missions followed by ground troops or radiation followed by tamoxifen, no one can really predict the outcome. We once warred against the Germans, the Japanese, and even Britain. Now they are our allies. While I can't conceive of cancer or the Taliban as an ally, I can picture a cease-fire. We'll never totally rout evildoers, but we can keep an eye on them in case they choose to activate. So America has its Homeland Security, and I have my "watchful waiting." Like someone on parole, I'll report periodically to the authorities and subject myself to careful scrutiny. Meanwhile, there is an ever-present threat that something, somewhere will pop out of the bushes like a Halloween goblin. We now live in a code red world. The president asks that we go about our lives as normally as possible. So, like everyone else, I'm on high alert but functioning as though everything is just fine. What a tribute to the adaptability of the human spirit.

Lost and Found

I am an artist, and I can't imagine myself doing anything else for a living. It's taken me many years, including having to deal with breast cancer, to come to that realization.

When I was a young wife and mother, I chose to put my family's interest and welfare ahead of mine. My husband traveled a lot with his job, and we were transferred often by the company for which he worked, so it was up to me to help settle Andrew and Emily, our two children, in new neighborhoods, schools, and activities over and over again. Because of the time and energy this took from me, I felt that I didn't have enough left over to do the artwork that I loved.

I fell in love with art at a young age. My mother was an artist, and she encouraged me to try my hand at it, too. I had chronic asthma and allergies when I was little and had to rest a lot. I would miss two weeks of school at a time, so art became my companion and salvation. I remember sitting on my bed, surrounded by my paints, constantly working on pictures and projects. My mom never minded all the bedsheets I stained with paint or piles of supplies that turned my bedroom into a studio. Once, after finally getting well enough to return to second grade, I informed my teacher that I would only be using my blue crayon for a while. Picasso had a "blue period" with his art, so I thought I would try it for now. Art became my identity.

It's no wonder that when I went away to college at Miami University in Oxford, Ohio, I majored in painting and graphic design, earning a bachelor's degree in fine arts. I fell in love and married my husband, Rob, after graduating and then worked in many advertising and graphic design studios to help pay the bills. The work was interesting, but it was many times less satisfying in a creative sense. When our children were born and all the moving started, I let my artistic pursuits be swept under the rug.

By the time our sixth move occurred, this one from the Chicago area to the Philadelphia area, I promised myself that no matter what, I would take an art class and get painting again. That wasn't the only thing on my mind, though, as we packed our bags and boxed our belongings. During a routine mammogram, calcifications had been found in my left breast, and I would need to repeat that mammogram in six months. I wasn't really worried about it because I knew that 90 percent of calcifications were not cancerous, and besides, I told myself, I was a low risk. I didn't have a strong family history of breast cancer; I ate relatively healthy, exercised regularly, and kept my weight down.

Unfortunately, a few months later in Philadelphia, a mammogram and biopsy revealed two separate cancerous tumors in my breast. When I received the news, I felt like I had been hit in the chest with a sledgehammer. I was numb and hardly functioning until I talked to my surgeon, who was out of town at the time, and he reassured me, "I just want you to know that you will not die from this." At that point I knew that I had hit bottom and was on my way up. I would just do whatever I needed to do to get well.

His reassuring words not only comforted me but also gave me the courage and determination to move from worry to action. I chose to have a double mastectomy because I didn't want to take the chance of it coming back in the other breast. I believed that doing everything I was offered was like taking out extra insurance policies to get rid of and prevent more cancer. I became very focused in my life's goals and priorities. I wanted to grow old with my husband, raise our two wonderful children, and once again do my artwork.

After all the surgery, I went through radiation because one tumor was 3 millimeters from my chest wall. And I followed with six months of chemotherapy and later tamoxifen. The recovery was slow and steady, but I was healed due to my age of 42, my supportive husband, family, and friends, my superior medical care, and especially that watercolor painting class I finally took. In addition, doctors gave me a 90 percent probability that I won't get breast cancer ever again!

Sometimes I feel that before I had breast cancer, I let the world around me dictate what I needed to be and do. I listened too much to the outside voices: eat less, exercise more, you are never too thin, work harder, volunteer even when you don't want to, do your part, strive for perfection (whatever that is), always give of yourself and take care of others even when you feel you can't. If you work at it hard enough, you can create a perfect little world and achieve eternal happiness.

After breast cancer, it was time for the real me to awaken. I started listening to my inner voices, which I believe come from my heart and soul. I took the time to meditate, do my artwork, and surround myself with the people who meant the most to me. One of my greatest accomplishments was learning how to say the word "No." I had a good excuse to stay on the sidelines when people asked for my time while I was going through chemotherapy or radiation. But after I recovered, I decided I didn't owe anyone an explanation about why I chose or did not choose to do something. I decided that the only volunteer work I would perform with my valuable time was when it would enable me to be with my children or it would directly affect them. It may sound selfish, but I've found that since I adopted this philosophy, I've been happier and less resentful, and I can accomplish more without feeling depleted. I'm satisfied knowing that I'm doing the best I can with what I have to work with.

I learned how to nourish myself and forgive myself for my imperfections. I found an inner peace that gave me creative energy and satisfaction. I was still able to give of myself and take care of my family and responsibilities, but I set limits and made time to renew my spirit. I prayed to God, "Please guide me in finding and fulfilling my purpose on earth. You gave me a wonderful talent, you got my attention with breast cancer—now open my mind and help direct me to change the rest of my life so that it can be fulfilling and not depleting."

> *I REALIZED HOW much I loved being an artist and painting again. It is a large part of my purpose and who I am. It's essential for my health, happiness, and sanity.*

Through that watercolor class, I found my lost talent, inner peace and purpose. I realized how much I loved being an artist and painting again. It is a large part of my purpose and who I am. It's essential for my health, happiness, and sanity.

Today, back in the Chicago area again, I do a variety of artwork for others and myself. I'm a decorative painter in people's homes, which includes painting wall murals, trompe l'oeil (a French term meaning "to fool the eye," in which, for example, realistic-looking flower-filled urns are painted on walls), and faux painting. Sometimes in the middle of a job a client will ask me, "How do you know what to do next?"

"I'm not sure," I tell them. "Sometimes painting feels like I'm channeling divine energy. I feel an almost out-of-body experience and a lightness and calmness wash over me."

I recently had a friend and client ask me how I could stand on my feet or up on a ladder all day and paint. I told her, "I'd rather do this than breathe."

It's such a wonderful feeling to have something from the inside come out and to share it with others and give them so much pleasure. It satisfies me, too, that my hand and brain created a painting others will look at and enjoy for a long, long time.

My main goal is to keep creating my art. I'd like to expand into the arena of children's books and maybe dabble with American primitive folk art. I have finally learned how important it is to listen to myself concerning what I need to nourish my soul. For me it is an integral part of healing and wellness.

The Gift

Y ou're what?" I gripped the phone tighter and waited for my daughter to say that she was kidding. Maybe I heard her wrong.

"I'm pregnant."

"Pregnant? But—"

"I know, I know. This is a surprise. Maybe you'll finally get that granddaughter you've been wanting."

I forced a positive note into my voice. "That would be . . . wonderful," I replied, but my daughter knew me too well.

"Mom, don't worry. Everything will be fine."

Everything will be fine. I had been clinging to that hope for the past few weeks while going for radiation treatments for breast cancer, but I wasn't really sure I believed it. And now this! Another worry.

I hung up the phone and felt a surge of panic. What was she thinking? She already had her hands full with three sons under the age of 10. Because she had her babies by C-section, her doctor warned her that another pregnancy would be risky. Worry and fear had been my constant companions of late, and I suddenly felt overwhelmed. My heart pounded with anxiety, and I wondered again why she hadn't been more careful. She was going to need me now more than ever. I had to be positive; I had to be strong.

It wasn't easy. The treatments made me tired and sore, and I hated the lines of worry etched on my husband's face. I just wanted the whole ordeal to go away, to be over. It was difficult not to be angry and not to question why this had to happen to me.

But as my daughter's tummy began to expand, so did my thinking. This baby represented life, hope, and a reason to face my fears and worries head-on.

I couldn't wait to hold this baby in my arms.

Finally, the day of her scheduled C-section arrived. I entered her house in the wee hours of the morning to watch the boys. "I love you," I said, giving her a tight hug before she got into the car.

"Mom, everything is going to be okay. We'll call you as soon as the baby is born."

I paced and prayed, staring at the phone, willing it to ring. When it finally did, I pounced on it. "Hello!"

"It's a girl!" Her voice was filled with joy. "A beautiful baby girl, and we've named her Cara."

"Oh, thank you! Thank you." My knees went weak with relief.

She laughed at my silly response. "You're welcome, Mom, but I think I should be thanking *you*."

"What?"

"You know this pregnancy was a total surprise."

"Yes, I do." I smiled, suddenly knowing what she was going to tell me—something I had suspected all along.

"When I found out you had breast cancer, I was really upset. I couldn't eat, couldn't sleep, and I really think this messed up my menstrual cycle. Believe me, there was no way I should have gotten pregnant. So, I'm thanking *you*, Mom. Thank you for my daughter."

As soon as I could, I rushed over to the hospital to see my new granddaughter. When I finally got to hold the tiny bundle in my arms, I beamed at my daughter. "She's beautiful."

"Spoken like a true grandmother," responded my daughter with a chuckle.

I ran a fingertip over the peachy softness of her cheek. I drank in the sight of her Cupid's bow mouth and perfect little nose, and I grinned at the pink bow taped onto her very little wispy blond hair. "You are my gift," I whispered in the tiny shell of her ear, and for the first time in many months, I experienced total joy.

Facing death had given me a whole new appreciation for the miracle of life.

Her birth in many ways was like a rebirth for me. Facing death had given me a whole new appreciation for the miracle of life.

That was 11 years ago, and I still think of Cara as my special gift. She was born nine months after I was diagnosed with cancer, and if my illness played a part in her birth, then I would gladly do it all over again. Since then, I have been given two more grandchildren, a total of nine, and another child is on the way. Ryan, John, Tim, Justin, Joe, David, Cara, Caroline, Jake, and baby, you are the light of my life, my hope, my joy, a precious gift, one and all.

Jeanne Rowe

Tune In to Your Emotions

I once heard a psychologist on the radio say that in a crisis a person should do three things: (1) talk about what she's feeling, (2) get the facts, and (3) make a plan of action. That sounded like good advice to me, and I took it to heart in dealing with breast cancer, which was diagnosed when I was 41 years old. For me, the biggest challenge on the radio psychologist's list was sharing my feelings about the diagnosis and the eventual lumpectomy, which had been a popular surgical procedure in Europe but was relatively new here in the United States.

I grew up during the "silent generation" of the 1940s and 1950s, when a roof over your head and food in your stomach were far more important than what you were thinking and feeling. Add to that the strict obedience expected from my parochial school teachers, and I became a girl who stayed out of trouble, who learned to do what she was supposed to do, and who kept her emotions tucked deep inside her being. That programming followed me into adulthood. Until breast cancer struck, I believed I should figure out my own problems rather than lay them on someone else. But you know what? I couldn't do that anymore when breast cancer was diagnosed. There were so many emotions and thoughts racing through my mind, about things like medical treatments, my mortality, and the uncertain future, that I didn't want to bury them because in one way or another, they would affect me. I also knew that they could possibly poison me. Instead, I believed that in order to heal, I had to talk to others and seek their support.

I thought a good place to start sharing the news about my breast cancer was at work, but some acquaintances and co-workers started avoiding me when they heard I had breast cancer. Sure, it hurt, but it was a good way to determine who really cared about me. And I found others, including family members, friends, and coworkers, who not only listened and offered help but also prayed for me. When I went into surgery, a group of coworkers at the mental health clinic held a "circle of light" for me. They gathered in a small room where they formed a circle, held hands, and focused on concentrating their collective energy and sending it to me as I lay on the operating table. That "light" is believed to aid healing, and all I can say is something must have worked right because the surgeon told me, "Your quick recovery is phenomenal!"

Finding a support group of other breast cancer survivors was also important to me because I wanted to be able to communicate with people who had some of the same experiences I did or who were about to face them. It wasn't easy to find the right fit, though. I did some research and found a group that, unfortunately, made me feel worse by the time I left than when I walked in with a smile and hopeful expectations. A hospital nurse facilitated the group of 15 people who gathered in a circle, some seated in stainless steel accented chairs and others in wheelchairs. When the participants introduced themselves and spoke at length about their medical treatments, I realized many of the people in the room were suffering from forms of cancer other than breast cancer and their prognosis for the future was bleak. When the depressing session was over, I caught up with about four breast cancer patients who were there, got their phone numbers, and invited each of them to form a new group, one we could call our own, to exchange ideas and feelings and to pursue a more positive outlook. I can't tell you how good it felt to share our hopes for the future, whether it was about breast cancer recovery or goals we had. "I want to live to see my son graduate from high school," I told my support group friends.

I remember Clare telling us, "I've always wanted to take a trip around the world, and now seems the time."

One of the support group members and I decided to attend a conference in Seattle called The Healing Power of Laughter and Play. Talk about allowing your emotions to come out and letting laughter become some of your best medicine! We drove five hours to that conference, where several hundred of us wore big red clown noses. It's hard to take anything seriously

I LEARNED THAT none of us is alone in our anxieties and that since we all have idiosyncrasies, we may as well laugh at them.

when the people around you look so goofy. We were prompted by mixer questions like "What's the ugliest present you ever got?" and "What's the most unusual job you ever applied for?"

After three days of playing, sharing thoughts, and laughing a lot, I learned that none of us is alone in our anxieties and that since we all have idiosyncrasies, we may as well laugh at them. I now believe that laughter is a tonic that can help reduce stress, alleviate pain, stimulate the immune system, and help improve the overall quality of life.

Thanks to my willingness to share my emotions, I've been a member of several support groups, and I've met the most incredible people from all walks of life—people I never would have met if it weren't for breast cancer. There was Jane, a quick-witted 72-year-old woman who loved to dress up as a clown and entertain at parties and nursing homes; Melody, a 37-year-old teacher who had cancer twice and was determined to see the world; Chris, a 29-year-old sensitive guy who had several types of experimental treatments and managed to beat the odds; and Tim, the 35-year-old father with malignant melanoma, who made a video for his seven-year-old daughter so she'd remember him after he was gone.

In the support group named Danica (which means "morning star" in Croatian), several of us met twice a month, shared a light supper, and opened our hearts to one another about our illnesses as we listened and offered hope. Our illnesses were viewed not as a tragedy but as a journey from which we would learn and experience all that life offered. Each meeting began and ended with hugs. At the end, we would form a circle where we would exchange spontaneous thoughts and prayers. A simple prayer I learned there is one I continue to say at least once a day:

> *The spirit of God lies within me.*
> *My mind and my body are at peace*
> *With this life within me.*
> *And I am healed.*

In addition to talking about my feelings, I took the radio psychologist's advice to get the facts. I learned that there are many avenues to healing and that the physical aspect is just one of them. I spent hours poring over books and journals trying to learn as much as I could about my illness so that I could ask doctors intelligent questions. Often I'd run into someone in a bookstore or health food store who would share treatment information, thereby giving me more hope.

One of my most valuable guides was a beautiful, soft-spoken Native American woman. "Slow down and listen to your body," she advised me. "See your disease as a telegram. Do not shoot the messenger, but simply take the message and gently send the messenger away."

That advice helped me form my plan of action beyond sharing my emotions. I decided that whether I lived or died, I would take care of myself and would make the most of my life. I now start my day looking in the mirror and saying, "I love you just the way you are."

I walk about a mile every day. I rest when I'm tired. I eat healthy foods like whole grains, foods with little sugar or fat, and I have lots of fruits and vegetables. Caffeine and alcohol are no longer a part of my diet. Every day I take a 20-minute break to pray and meditate, and I've learned that there is no room for negative people in my valuable life. The rewards have been bountiful! The cancer has been gone for 20 years. I feel healthier mentally and physically. The migraines that plagued me for seven years disappeared, and I lost 20 pounds.

I no longer live a life of predictability but instead live one of passion. You can find me skipping my routine from time to time when I visit a garden, peruse a card or bookstore (often checking out the humor section), or stop by a park to ride on a swing. More often than not, I'll be visiting with a stranger, talking, and as you've probably guessed, expressing my emotions.

Breast cancer has taught me that what I think and feel is important and there's no reason to tune out my thoughts, which is just what the radio psychologist prescribed.

Walking in the Winter Wilderness

Okay," says Sally to the women lined up in the winter night. We have struggled to get our snowshoes on and are waiting apprehensively for what comes next. "Take one step forward," Sally commands, then pauses as we tentatively move ahead a pace.

"Congratulations!" she announces with a grin. "You are now intermediate snowshoers."

This is a very special night. Our diverse group of about a hundred women is gathered at Eagle Mountain, a cross-country ski area in California's Sierra Nevada.

We're here for a Full Moon Snow Shoe Hike sponsored by Sally Edwards and Melissa McKenzie, cofounders of YubaShoes, a company that makes sports snowshoes. The hike is a memorial to their mothers, who both died of breast cancer, and a fund-raiser for the Breast Cancer Fund.

Each of the hikers has a connection to breast cancer. Some are involved through their own health, others because of a friend or relative. I'm connected through my dad's mother, who ultimately died of natural causes nearly 40 years after radical surgery in the late 1940s, and my mom's younger sister, who succumbed to cancer at the age of 80.

The night is cold but windless. In the west, Venus blazes like a torch in the sky. To the east, an orange sherbet full moon is just clearing the snowy mountains. We're in an enormous silent cathedral with an endless ceiling of brilliant stars, and we find ourselves speaking in murmurs, unwilling to shatter the magical calm of the night.

As we head out through a frigid forest of naked trees, their branches as black as ink, our eyes are fixed on our feet. Left, right. Actually the snowshoes aren't so tough. Left, right. We can really do this. Left, right. Yes, we are walking easily, powerfully, buoyantly on the snow.

We become more aware of our surroundings. Higher in the sky now, the moon gleams silver—so bright that we leave our flashlights in our pockets. The trees throw shadows like calligraphy across the trail and the metal cleats on our snowshoes scratch almost musically against the snow's light crust. The icy air smells alive somehow, and the snow, sampled from a mitten, tastes pure and clean.

Our long line gradually coalesces into small groups with conversations growing. What's your name? Where are you from? Have you ever done this before?

Finally, we emerge onto a wide meadow where the snow glistens like sugar in the moonlight.

We make our way around the meadow and gather around a bonfire burning vigorously atop a large piece of metal. (Without the metal, of course, the fire could extinguish itself as it melts the snow.)

Sally welcomes us, then says, "Let's get acquainted. As we go around the circle, give your name and who you are. I don't mean what you do," she cautions. "I mean the 'who.' This is very hard for some people."

We sit, watching the fire, its orange, yellow, and red flames blossoming against the black-and-white night. We don't look at each other.

Finally, Sally says, "Okay, I'll start. I'm an athlete and my mission in life is getting people fit. When people get in tune with their bodies, the rest of their lives can start working for them. I like to ask people, 'When is the last time you did something for the first time?'"

"Tonight!" someone exclaims, and almost all of us raise our mittened hands proudly. We are women together doing something new and physical and special.

After a moment, another woman introduces herself and recites a poem she wrote in her mind as she tramped through the snow. The woman next to her, abruptly widowed, speaks of the importance of women friends over 25 years.

"I'm a writer," I say. "I guess it's both who I am and what I do." I see stories everywhere, I explain—including this hike—and want to write those stories so other people can see them, too.

It's fascinating hearing from these women who are strangers, yet already friends. Single, married, widowed, divorced. An attorney, a college student, a young mother, a high school teacher, an entrepreneur.

Some are struggling with breast cancer, a death, losing a job, the end of a marriage, or just plain life. One, formerly a schoolteacher, is now a stay-at-home mother. "Sally wants us to say who we are," she muses, "but I'm not sure anymore except I'm a mom. Right now I don't even have the energy to find out who else I am."

Another confides that she's going through a big crisis since breast cancer forced her to leave her job. "I'd always been what I did, but now I'm not anymore. I don't want to be all about cancer, but it's taking up most of my life right now. I'm struggling to find out who I am."

"Can I just go straight to the crisis part?" asks another in a weary tone. She's also been coping with breast cancer, but as she speaks her voice takes on life. "This year has been awful and wonderful. There are lot of people coming into my life—mostly women—so there is good that came from the crisis."

"Today is the one year anniversary of my cancer surgery," says another, and the circle breaks into applause, muffled by our mittens and gloves. "I didn't know if I'd make it. I sure didn't know I'd be here."

"I'm a grandmother," says another, gesturing at her two teenaged granddaughters who have accompanied her. Her voice takes on a tone of awe. "I never worked outside the home. I never went out alone at night. And here I am in the wilderness."

Being out in the moonlight and snow is such an accomplishment for every one of us that it's nearly impossible to describe. We are jubilant. We are triumphant. We are strong.

Although we're becoming chilled, there is a real reluctance to let go of this magical time. Being out in the moonlight and snow is such an accomplishment for every one of us—a thrill, a satisfaction, an achievement—that it's nearly impossible to describe. We are jubilant. We are triumphant. We are strong. And we all feel an extraordinary bond.

But finally we head back across the meadow, gathering again in the lodge, where refreshments and a roaring fire await. "What was it like?" Sally asks, and this time everyone is eager to offer a comment.

"I like to do things I've never done before," declares one woman. "I like to take risks—not stupid risks, but things that are a challenge, and this was a challenge."

Another woman, whose children are grown, says, "This is the best time of my life. I think women know how to play exquisitely—cooperatively instead of competitively. The physical, like snowshoeing in the dark, doesn't come naturally to me, but when I master it, I have such a strong sense of personal power."

"I felt an incredible sense of accomplishment," echoes another, "and a wonderful sense of myself."

"It was easier than I thought it would be," another woman says, "and it was incredibly wonderful. The most peaceful serenity. It's absolutely one of the neatest things I've ever done."

"To be around a campfire with a lot of women was one of the high points of my life," chimes in another. "This is something I'm going to cherish."

"I'm overwhelmed," another woman says, shaking her head in wonder. "Overwhelmed in a very good way. Struggling with cancer, I've had to be so tough, and I am so tired of being so tough. I've had trouble finding strong women, and here you all are."

"Campfires and women together like this are very powerful," agrees Sally. "It's special doing something for the first time. There's energy, adventure, and women triumphing together."

Cancer Compelled Me to Follow My Dreams

For your first wedding anniversary, you're supposed to receive paper presents, so when ours rolled around, I was hoping for a gift certificate to our favorite B&B, tickets to *Les Miz,* or the latest Sue Grafton mystery.

Instead, I got breast cancer.

Not exactly a gift that can be returned, although I tried.

It was just a week earlier when I'd accidentally felt something in my left breast while lying in bed, engrossed in my Agatha Christie. I'd reached up to push my hair out of my eyes when my hand grazed my breast—in itself a miracle, 'cause I'm not Dolly Parton to start with, and lying down, I have the chest of a 10-year-old girl—and I touched something that felt like a hard pea.

Like many women, I have fibrocystic, or "lumpy," breasts so I wasn't too worried about it. But just to be safe, the next day, I called my doctor for an appointment. When she examined me, she wasn't too concerned either, thinking it might simply be the result of too much caffeine or probably a water-filled cyst. However, just to be on the safe side, she scheduled a mammogram.

And I'm glad she did.

Thankfully, I'd had a baseline mammogram two years earlier, when I was 33, which I had insisted upon because of a lump I'd felt at the time, combined with a family history of breast cancer (my mom). When the latest mammogram came back, it showed a difference from the baseline. Because of that difference, I'm here today.

I was so thankful for that mammogram that I wrote a little song (sung to the tune of "Thanks for the Memory") to express my gratitude:

> *Thanks for the mammogram.*
> *A small squish goes a long way*
> *To finding the Big C.*
> *It really can help save the life*
> *Of folks like you and me.*
> *Get your mam-mogram!*

What can I say? I'm a musical kind of gal. And since I never made it to Broadway, this is my opportunity.

The difference in mammograms prompted the doctor to order a biopsy. My husband, Michael, and I weren't worried about it—I really thought everything would be fine, no problem—but just in case, I didn't want it to mar our first wedding anniversary. So we scheduled the biopsy for the day after.

August 5, 1992, we learned I had breast cancer.

I was 35 years old, had *finally* gotten my college degree three months before after years of stopping and starting, and was at long last married to the soul mate I'd been looking for my entire life.

How could I lose it all now?

I didn't.

All I "lost" were a breast, some lymph nodes, my hair (temporarily), and 30 unwanted pounds on the original Slim-Fast chemo diet.

Cancer affects every woman differently. Some women struggle with the thought of losing a breast, and feeling like less of a woman. Or they worry how their husbands will respond to them. Others regret the loss of their luxuriant mane of crowning glory.

My "luxuriant mane" lasted for about a two-year permed period in my late 20s. Other than that, it had always been rather short and on the thin side, so hair loss wasn't a big deal to me, especially since I knew it would grow back.

And my breasts have always been on the thin—small—side, too (the only thing on my body that is), so there wouldn't be much to miss in that department either. Besides, God gave me a wonderful loving husband (after making me wait what seemed like an eternity for him) who, when he first saw my mastectomy scar, kissed it and said, "I love this scar because it means I'm going to have you with me for a long time."

So I didn't struggle in those areas.

Chemotherapy was the toughest thing for me. I'd elected to participate in a National Cancer Institute clinical trial that was trying to prove that more intensive chemo in a shorter period of time was more effective. Participants in the study were given varying doses of chemotherapy, chosen randomly by computer. I was selected to get the heaviest dosage possible. My faith knows it wasn't "random," however. I got the dose I needed.

Unfortunately, the nurse at the hospital forgot to give me my anti-nausea medication before the first dose was ever administered, thus setting off a vicious cycle of nausea that caused me to retch every couple hours for 10 days straight. But on the up side, I did lose 30 pounds in 30 days!

After one of the treatments, when I'd returned home and Michael and I were snuggling in bed, he felt something strange and grew concerned.

"What *is* that, honey?" he asked.

"My hipbone!" I said joyfully.

I always try to look for the positive—or goofy—in any situation. I think that's what helped me get through my cancer experience. That, and God.

Many people ask "Why me?" when something like this befalls them. But I always thought "Why not me?" Why should I be exempt? Everything happens for a reason. Although we can't always see what that reason is, I can honestly say that cancer changed my life for the better, and I'm grateful for it.

> *I CAN HONESTLY say that cancer changed my life for the better, and I'm grateful for it.*

My encounter with breast cancer helped me to dust off a long-neglected dream—a dream I'd had since I read 103 books in Miss Vopelinsky's first-grade class: to be an author someday.

Five years after I discovered I had breast cancer, my first book was published—at the age of 40. A couple years later, I wrote the book of my heart, *Thanks for the Mammogram!* (Revell, 2000), to offer hope and encouragement to other women going through breast cancer. I now travel around the country speaking to women about my cancer experience and am also writing my seventh book. Although I'm going through "mentalpause" (another one of my book titles), my life is just beginning.

Art from the Heart, Year 5 *A.B.C.*

arch 27, 1998. Three days before my daughter's
12th birthday. It's the date I was first diagnosed.
It's since become the date from which I seem to
measure every event: either it happened B.B.C. (before breast
cancer) or A.B.C.

Living A.B.C. (happily ever after, one hopes) for me often
means trying to do whatever anyone with any authority sug-
gests might help me recover and stay healthy, even though
there is so little that anyone can suggest with certainty.

I try to eat right, even though professional dietitians say
there is no diet proven to prevent recurrence; most doctors
and magazine articles agree that low fat and lots of fruits and
vegetables is the best way to go, so that's the way I go.

I try to take it easy physically, especially since that
dreaded recurrence did occur, despite my dietary devotion. In
the spring of 2000, pain in my lower ribs, which my primary
care physician's associate first diagnosed as a clinical frac-
ture, turned out to be metastasized breast cancer. A CAT

scan in the emergency room revealed five spots in my liver and severe damage to the ribs and pelvis.

But the best advice I've taken is some I gave myself in the last two years—to spend however many days, months, or years I have left doing what I truly love to do.

Following my recovery from 1998's mastectomy, then chemotherapy and radiation treatments that lasted nearly a year, I tried to return to work full-time as my husband's partner in our public relations business. We'd built Jane and Ed Goldman Communications, Inc. into one of the 25 top PR firms in California's capital city of Sacramento, and I wasn't about to leave my partner in the lurch by pulling away from my responsibilities. But Ed, who'd already been simply the best husband and caretaker anyone could have wished for, reminded me that my life was mine to live, however I saw fit. And if I saw that as not being a full partner any longer, then he would pick up the slack.

But the best advice I've taken is some I gave myself—to spend however many days, months, or years I have left doing what I truly love to do.

He's not only picked up the slack, but he's kept the business going at an even stronger pace, with me providing advice and ideas and brainstorming as needed. And I've been able to at last pursue my dream of a full-time career making art.

I thank my lucky stars every day that I'm not only still alive but free to live that life to the fullest. I had attempted some painting B.B.C. with mild success. After years spent in high-powered jobs in the media and public relations, ranging from reporting and anchoring at a local top-rated network TV affiliate to managing public affairs for the Governor's

Office of Planning and Research, I gave birth, at the age of 35, to Jessica in 1986.

Again, thanks to Ed's generosity, I was able to spend the first five years of our daughter's life staying at home taking care of her. Whenever she napped, I hightailed it to a tiny studio off the dining room and built a body of figurative-narrative work that was shown in a number of prestigious galleries and restaurants around California.

I am largely self-taught, as were some of my greatest influences, including Van Gogh and Rousseau. I had wanted to paint since my college years at Northwestern University, where I was exposed to Chicago's Imagist/Hairy Who movement. That movement and my studies in journalism and psychology inspired the irreverent and humorous world view of my early figurative-narrative work. While I was pregnant with Jessica and during her early years, I took a few courses in drawing and painting, learning how to use color to create an emotional impact and tell a story.

My ever-larger and ever-brighter acrylic canvases expressed a deepening love for life but didn't sell particularly well. So once Jessica entered grade school, I decided I needed to return to the workaday world and make a stronger financial contribution to our family's well-being. I took a public relations job with the local electric utility for a year and a half, then joined Ed in the PR firm he'd founded in 1982. We worked hard and prospered, but my painting fell by the wayside.

Then came March 27, 1998. Faced with the harsh reality that my future was far from guaranteed, I came to appreciate the value of stopping to smell—and paint—the flowers.

When I was diagnosed and had surgery, so many people sent flowers to make me feel better. What's really ironic is, I'm allergic to flowers. My husband got a big table, set it up on the deck outside the kitchen window, and put all those gorgeous bouquets on it. And I photographed them. There was so much love in them. They made me feel so good. When I started painting again, I tried to capture the beauty of those flowers, with the hope that maybe my art would make people feel as good.

Changing my focus from fauna to flora began as a way to immortalize the feelings contained in each of those well-wishing blooms. Rather than lamenting the transitory nature of life, in the tradition of still-life painting, I wanted my paintings to celebrate the immortal nature of love. I chose oil, painting's longest-enduring medium, to capture and convey the indomitability of beauty. I used heavy-duty square canvases, some measuring as small as 5 inches by 5 inches, others 4 feet by 4 feet, to capture a single bloom in all its glory, with vibrant color wrapping around all four thick sides. Each canvas has a story to tell, with nature speaking through me. And since it's difficult to contemplate nature without becoming happier, I feel that these flowers have the power to comfort those who view them. One sees nature through one's own temperament: I believe that life, like flowers, can stay fresh forever. That's why I call them my "Power Flowers."

Often people who've survived disasters and catastrophic diseases talk about the miracle of the everyday, their new-found ability to find inspiration in the life around them daily. It's become a cliché; and frankly, I'd appreciated life before all of this happened. I didn't need this. Yet life now does have an added poignancy or power. When you're faced with the fact that you might not have the time you thought you would, you want to make every second count. Creating and sharing these paintings has brought me immeasurable hope and emotional healing.

When four fractures in my pelvis early in 2002 made painting large canvases a bit difficult, I simply funneled my appreciation for nature into a smaller format, creating one-of-a-kind art-to-wear jewelry pieces I call Janestones, which are made with the earth's natural ingredients—large gemstones, gold, silver, and ceremonial beads from all around the world.

Thanks to the miracle of modern medicine, my family and my faith, and my art, I've never given up for one second. I've never dropped the confidence that I'll prevail.

What I'm trying to do with my artwork is somehow help people feel the same joy I've felt in creating it. Just being alive and having the next day to look forward to is a miracle for me. I want to pass that on to people. I feel lucky. Very lucky.

It's as simple as A.B.C.

Whitney Sherman

Creating the Breast Cancer Research Stamp

W hen people learn that I created the Breast Cancer Research Stamp, they often ask if I'm a breast cancer survivor. Although I do not claim that experience, I did interview several survivors, including art director Ethel Kessler, as part of my research. We talked mostly about the importance of evoking hope, for the survivor and her family and friends, and about the nature of courage. I wondered how I could show hope in light of such a life-altering experience. How could I communicate the humanity (women, men, families) involved?

I remember staring at a blank page, pencil in hand, as I began to draw images I thought demonstrated spirit, strength, and courage—active bodies reaching up in triumph. I thought of the race in research to find a cure and the small victories that count. But the story of breast cancer is larger than life, and I felt challenged, even frustrated, by the complexity of making an image that works well in such a limited amount of space. As I contemplated my sketches, the same thought kept coming to me. Something is missing. Where is the heroic nature of the women, their caregivers, the doctors, and the researchers who are all involved in the fight against breast cancer?

The format of the stamp was such a small canvas on which to work. I knew that I had to carefully pick a subject, the gesture, the colors to portray a hopeful, positive message. The ideas behind the image needed to be strong. Showing a woman is best for that role, I decided. She would need to represent all ages, all races. How to show heroic? I instantly thought of mythology, especially Artemis, the huntress! She is an icon of independence and strength. She determines her own path and takes charge.

> ❧ SHE IS AN ICON OF *independence and strength. She determines her own path and takes charge.*

I thought of the quiver and arrow, ready to take aim. I drew her arm raised over her head, her profile facing right to represent the future, a place of hope, and wrapped her other arm around her waist, to hold the bow and frame her torso. Then I realized that she's in the position every woman assumes to prepare for a self-examination or mammogram! Artists call these occurrences happy accidents.

Satisfied with the sketch, I carried it to my photocopier to enlarge the image onto high-quality drawing paper. By being enlarged, the pencil marks looked more interesting. For the stamp, I used my pastels, colorful soft chalk, which I keep in a brown wooden box in a drawer. As I looked at the disarray of colorful sticks, I saw a riot of shapes and shades, each stick having been rubbed into a unique shape from work on previous pictures. They reminded me of the uniqueness of each woman battling breast cancer. As I looked at the many colors, I realized that using a specific skin tone would exclude someone. The figure needed to speak to all women because cancer does not discriminate. I decided to create a kaleido-scope of colors radiating out from the figure. Inspired by the radiant paintings of Chagall, I marked the paper with yellow, blue, orange, and green pastels, creating contrasts in broad, controlled strokes to the figure on the paper before me. I wanted the stamp to show colors that are both active and restful. I blended the pastels to achieve different densities, ul-timately creating a pattern of colors that are not separated from each other by borders or edges.

When I created the Breast Cancer Research Stamp in 1998, I didn't stop to contemplate the effect it would have. Now I am in awe of how it has affected people in so many ways. The sale of the stamp has raised enormous funds to support a collective effort to find answers to the lingering question of the potential cure. Aside from my obvious pride in creating the award-winning Breast Cancer Research Stamp, I feel a deep connection to the people who have come to meet me at signings, have shaken my hand, and have thanked me for making this stamp for them. That is truly an affirmation of the power of art to open doors in our hearts, minds, and souls. Art helps us to see more of the beauty around us, inspires us, and touches us in profound ways. And, in the end, it makes all of us better for the experience.

My hope is that the Breast Cancer Research Stamp will continue to inspire people to fund the fight far into the future and that it can remain a beacon of hope for a cure.

Marlys Thompson

Miracles Can Happen

Someone once said, "Your mind is like a bad neighborhood—don't go in there alone!" I can certainly identify with that! When I hear bad or scary news, my mind becomes consumed by it, and the information rolls around in my head, collecting more fear as it rolls, like a giant snowball. Before I know it, the bad or scary news is all I can think about.

That's what happened seven years ago when I went to the surgeon's office to get the results of a needle biopsy. We were sitting across from each other as he leaned over his large, brown, wooden desk toward me.

"Mrs. Thompson, you have cancer," he said matter-of-factly.

"*What???* They say that to *other* people," I thought to myself, as I heard him continue.

"It's relatively small. We can probably handle it with one surgery—a lumpectomy," he said.

"Do whatever you have to," was my sullen reply.

Three days later, I'm coming out of surgery, and I can tell by the look of disappointment on my surgeon's face that the results aren't good. "We were not able to get all of the cancer. One of the lymph nodes is infected. There's a high probability that it's spread. We recommend a mastectomy," he said.

His words still echo in my mind—even after seven years. I remember his tone. How serious he was.

How scared I was. It was too much for me to handle. "Can we talk about this tomorrow?" I managed to ask.

Even though I felt so overwhelmed about the possibility of having a mastectomy, somewhere between that moment and the next morning, I became clear and focused on one thought: "This is the body I came in with and this is the body I'm goin' out with." It became a mantra, a declaration—a place to focus. It gave me something to hang on to, repeating it over and over as I went forward. What did I mean by that mantra? In other words, "This is the package and the parts that God gave me, and I'm keeping them until I die of old age. I don't want a surgeon to change my body. It's the only one I have, and I want to keep her healthy and whole." To make that happen, I knew I needed every possible resource. I couldn't face this alone. I wasn't going to rely just on medical intervention. I needed to investigate other avenues of healing, and that meant finding others who could help. That snowball of fear was bigger than ever in my mind, and I didn't want it to keep rolling and collecting even more. Taking action was the only way to prevent that from happening.

The next morning, I called the surgeon and informed him, "I acknowledge you're a fine group of physicians"—and they were—"but I'm choosing to find some way my body can be healthy and whole. What's the maximum time you can give me before I have to make that decision?"

"Three weeks, and you're pushing it," was his disheartened reply.

Whew! Time to get movin'. I took this healing project on like an intense business venture. I did things I'd *never* done before. I worked with a nutritionist I had previously met at a meeting for small business owners. I traveled to her town 90 miles away. We met at her home. She covered some basic nutritional concepts and showed me a videotape. Then we visited a huge health food store. As we stood in the entryway of the store, my skepticism was apparent by the frown on my face. "I know there's a lot of good stuff in here," I said. "And I also know some of it tastes like cardboard. So can you guide me to some tasty food that's also healthy?"

As we pushed the silver metal shopping cart down the aisle, Sarah steered me toward fresh vegetables, wholesome grains like brown rice, different kinds of wheat-free pasta, bottled sauces and sugar-free dressings, frozen fish, and cooking items like a steamer pot and nonstick frying pans. And there were lots of fresh zesty spices and herbs to perk things up just the way I like it. As we shopped, we talked about how certain foods can boost my immune system and make my body stronger for the impending surgery, which continued to be a possibility and it lingered in my mind.

Sarah was also a great resource for others who could help me improve my health. She referred me to Susan, who was a "hands-on healer." My first visit was a disaster. Susan asked me to get in touch with my own internal wisdom. Huh? (The only wisdom I had was that my mind wasn't always my best friend.) I'd never done this before, so I fantasized what I'd do to find it. As a former private pilot, I pictured in my mind's eye a scanner, like some sort of infrared device that the army, or photographers, use at nighttime to see hidden objects. Only I used it to go inside my body. So I'm "scanning" inside my body—first the left leg, then the right one, then my left arm, and my torso, and finally the inside of my right arm. And then it happened. I started to giggle. I couldn't help it.

Susan asked, "What do you see?"

"I'm looking for my own internal wisdom . . . and nobody's home!" I said.

She was kind of serious and I was very nervous, feeling like I'd never get the hang of this inner wisdom stuff. Susan suggested, "I think that's enough for today. Let's try it again tomorrow."

The next day, Susan and I tried it again. And this time, I *was* able to see something. She placed her hands directly on the location where the cancer had been found, and she mentally and verbally walked me through several very calming, healing visualizations. "Picture this part of your body as being healthy and whole," she coaxed me. It felt very good to have someone be so loving, and so comforting, and so focused just on me. By the time I left that session, I felt more at peace with myself and like I wasn't alone in this battle.

The hands-on healing also helped me feel closer to God. I prayed at another level. Prior to the cancer, I would pray from time to time. Mostly, it was when I needed something or when I was frustrated that I couldn't figure out something. During the hands-on healing experience, Susan had me picture Jesus placing his hands on the top of my head. As he placed his hands on my head, my whole body was filled with white healing light. I would breathe deeply in and out as the light moved from the top of my head to fill my body cavity, pausing and focusing where the cancer had been found, and

To this day, my mornings begin with prayers of gratitude, and my evenings conclude the same way. It gives me peace.

then moving on down throughout my body, until it reached the tip of my toes.

Somehow after doing that so frequently during the day (and also every night), I just felt so much closer to a divine spirit that I would speak freely as if I were talking to my best buddy—only with a little more reverence. My prayers and conversations with God occurred much more frequently. And even today, whenever possible, I'll look at something in nature, like a tree (outside a building or outside my car), as I speak to God and express gratitude and/or ask for help for myself, a friend, or some member of my family. I just feel so blessed and so much more connected—not alone. I'm part of nature. And God's wonder is reflected there for me.

To this day, my mornings begin with prayers of gratitude, and my evenings conclude the same way. It gives me peace.

I also talked with people about mind-body connection. I learned of a study from Harvard in 1979, by psychologist Ellen Langer and her colleagues. The premise of the experiment was that the aging process is directly influenced by whether a person sees himself as old or young. (I thought that maybe it could work with my fight against cancer, but instead of old or young, it would be healthy or sick.) The researchers invited a group of men who were 75 years old and older to a weeklong retreat; the clock was turned back to 1959, when all of them were 20 years younger and more vibrant. For example, the only music they heard was from 20 years earlier. They read magazines from 1959 and were instructed to talk about events and people they remembered from the 1950s. The results of this experiment were incredibly inspiring. Researchers found the men had an increase in memory, improved manual dexterity, and more flexible joints, and their posture had started to improve. What impressed me most was the fact that the length of their fingers (which tend to contract due to age) had actually extended—in only a week!

Mind over matter. Sounded like it could work for me.

My head was swimming with all of the information I collected over the few weeks I had. Many times I was in a state of feeling overwhelmed. I knew I couldn't keep it all straight in my head. So I created a binder with all the notes from all the conversations and all the conclusions that occurred as I went from one step of the journey to the next one. On the front of the binder, I wrote, "MY BODY IS HEALTHY & WHOLE." And I just looked at those words . . . over, and over, and over again.

At the end of three weeks, it was time to go back to my surgeon. He looked incredulous as I said, "I don't think the cancer's there anymore."

"Can you be sure?" he asked.

I told him about all the different healing avenues I had taken and told him, "I can't be 100 percent sure because some of this stuff could be, what I call, California woo-woo, but something inside tells me I'm right."

He was somewhat skeptical—but still willing to listen. I asked him, "What's the possibility of you going in there and just taking a little 'scoop' to check it out? And I'll go along with whatever you find."

"Well, it'll cost you for two operations," he said.

"That's okay with me," I responded.

And to make a long story short, when they went in, the cancer had disappeared. It disappeared!

It disappeared! I was blessed to understand at a cellular level—at my basic core—the power of shifting my perspective of what's possible, putting structures in place to support what I want to have happen, and working with other people in *new* ways. None of that would have been possible if I'd limited myself and stayed in my own mind. There were no resources there—it was only filled with fear, big time. I had to go "outside the neighborhood."

After the cancer had "disappeared," the doctors still recommended I go through radiation and chemotherapy. It was time to get a second opinion. A colleague from the San Francisco area (who also had cancer) referred me to another surgeon. I made an appointment and took a friend with me to help me remember what to ask and to record his responses. This surgeon was not a fan of chemotherapy because he believed it did a body more harm than good. He looked me straight in the eye and said, "Only *you* can decide. How will you feel if you don't do chemo and 10 years from now it comes back and people say to you, 'Boy, were you stupid'? And how will you feel if 15 years from now you're still cancer-free, and people say, 'Boy, were you lucky'?"

I just knew that this body wasn't strong enough to have chemotherapy, so I decided against it. I did do the radiation every day for seven weeks, though.

Fast-forward to seven years later. I've joined a nine-year study through the University of California where researchers are looking at the impact of nutrition on diminishing the recurrence of cancer. Those people have been a godsend because they've taught me so much about nutrition. For example, I never knew anything about carrot juice. Now I have a glass every day. The phytochemicals in vegetable juice are thought to be disease inhibitors for cancer, and you're able to absorb a larger volume through juicing rather than eating the whole vegetable. Besides that, I just *feel* good when I drink it—clean and healthy. It's kind of hard to describe, but it's true. I've taken cooking classes, from the University of California people from the Davis campus, on how to easily prepare tasty, low-fat, nutritious meals. (Another reward is that I've met other women who have had breast cancer, and we share more than recipes.)

At one point of the study, a university nutritionist from the San Diego campus called each week to see how I was doing with my menu planning and preparation and to ask if I had any questions. Over time, the calls shifted to once every other week, then once a month. And now it's once a quarter—every three months. I fax her my "food recall" for the week before. It's always a great reminder to keep myself on track. She enters the information into her computer. It calculates all the different elements of amount of fat, carbohydrates, proteins, salts, and so forth. And we talk and she still teaches me. I also go to a local facility for different blood tests, urine tests, blood pressure, and whatever else they want to measure so they can establish different benchmarks. There's no cost. They're happy I'm still participating in the study. I'm happy they're still teaching me.

> *Breast cancer has taught me that I am the author of my life and that I'm not in this life alone.*

Before the cancer, I wouldn't have even noticed or been conscious of what this body needs. Now I'm so thankful that she's still working, that I do my best to listen. What do I really want and need in this moment, physically *and* emotionally? And what actions do I need to take to make it happen?

Breast cancer has taught me that I am the author of my life and that I'm not in this life alone. I have other people to add dimension, learning, and joy to my life. Two heads are better than one. Heartfelt joys, as well as fears, are better when shared. Miracles can happen. I'm living proof.

Ramona Catherine Murray de Prieto

We Are All Connected

Being part of one of the most outstanding law enforcement agencies in the world gives its members a common thread. As the first female California Highway Patrol motorcycle officer, I had the honor of being part of an elite group, the central Los Angeles motorcycle officers contingent. I may not have fit the typical stereotype of a motorcycle officer, but I was so proud to be a part of that team. To me, getting that job was about setting a goal, charting a course, and realizing what I needed to do to impact my options for life.

That's exactly what I had to do 20 years later when I found a lump in my left breast while taking a shower. I was demonstrating a breast self-exam to my daughters, five-year-old Nina and 11-year-old Ramona, to share with them information that I had just learned at a women's health fair. As I demonstrated the newly learned technique, to my surprise, I felt a lump the size of a tiny pea.

When I called my doctor, the office related that since I'd had a mammogram a month ago, there was probably little reason to worry, but they said they could schedule some tests. "I'd like to get some tests done immediately," I responded.

A breast ultrasound led to a needle biopsy, and before I knew it, I was listening to a surgeon asking me, "Do you want me to take out your left breast or just remove the lump?"

I felt like a cement truck had just dumped its load on me. Throughout the tests each practitioner was hopeful and reassuring, so I wasn't adequately prepared for the conversation with the surgeon. After telling the doctor I'd prefer a lumpectomy, I got into my car and sobbed, not only for myself but for my daughters, who I feared might grow up without a mother. "Who will care for them if I'm gone?" I wondered.

Law enforcement trains a person to control her emotions, using the brain over emotions. Yet nothing in law enforcement training could keep me from my intense feelings of anguish over how my potential death would impact my children. During that time more than ever, I believed it was the inner strength nourished by great friends, family, and God that carried me through those tough times.

The first surgery revealed that instead of having just one lump, I had six. As I was awakening from the first surgery, the surgeon related that she wanted to perform a mastectomy. It was too much information to handle at that time, so I put off a decision. Instead, I regrouped, charted my course, and looked at my options.

Going to the University of California at Los Angeles Revlon Breast Center for a second opinion was the best decision I could have made for my family and myself. I spoke to five specialists for four hours, and together they came up with a multifaceted plan to deal with the type of breast cancer I had. I ended up going through six lumpectomies that eventually led to a mastectomy because all of the cancer could not be removed.

When word about my breast cancer spread throughout the California Highway Patrol family, I received more than 200 get well cards, and two to three bouquets of flowers or plants arrived every day. At one point, there were 62 living plants in our home, thriving and growing healthier. I felt embraced and inspired by the close-knit California Highway Patrol family and was encouraged to be a strong fighter for life.

All of the visits, phone calls, cards, and flowers not only helped me see the connection that we all share, but it also made me see that together we could make it through the journey.

The phone calls, cards, and gifts showed me that we're all connected. When I was feeling like breast cancer was the end of the world and I was all alone, my friends and colleagues became guardian angels, carrying me to a new level. Some came to visit weekly to pray with me, and that helped me draw on their strength. All of the visits, phone calls, cards, and flowers not only helped me see the connection that we all share, but it also took a heavy load off of my shoulders and made me see that together we could make it through the journey.

That's why I'm so open about sharing what I have learned about a new perspective and breast cancer. When a good friend suggested that I be interviewed for the first article creating awareness of breast cancer in a California Highway Patrol publication, I was honored to be a part of it. If I can help just one person and make a difference in her life, that's what it's all about. When you are stricken by a life-threatening illness, you can't help but feel passionate about it and wonder how you can make a positive impact in the lives of others.

When I accept invitations to give speeches about breast cancer to women's groups, I tell them that I was lucky to find my breast cancer so early. "You could be one of the lucky ones, too," I say, "if you remember to check your breasts each month. Contact the American Cancer Society at (800) 227-2345 to get a plastic breast self-exam shower card."

I also urge the audience to buy breast cancer postage stamps to fund research. "Buy one less mocha a week and you can afford the stamps," I offer.

Sometimes when my telephone rings, it's a call from a woman who has been diagnosed with breast cancer and who got my name through the grapevine. At first the conversation can be a little awkward, so I tell her what happened to me and add, "It was like climbing a mountain; I took one step at a time and immersed myself in information and exceptional medical care."

I refer her to helpful Internet sites and advise her to get a jogging bra that hooks in the front. It helps hold bandages in place after surgery. "Before you lose your hair, go buy a wig, some comfortable hats or wraps, and buy some big earrings to dress it up," I add.

When I share what I've learned with others who are feeling so alone and desperate, it helps me realize how blessed I was with my extended family and friends and clearly shows me how we are all connected.

One of my favorite sayings has brought me comfort over the years and especially during my journey and crisis. It's from Martin Luther King, Jr., who said, "The ultimate measure of a [person] is not where [she] stands in moments of comfort and convenience, but where [she] stands at times of challenge and controversy."

The challenge for me was the disease and how to deal with that disease; the controversy came from the different treatment methods suggested by the different doctors and the level of information interchange by all involved. The controversy went beyond selecting the best treatment for my condition—it also encompassed digesting what the experts had to say and the information presented or withheld. I chose to stand up, fight the disease, and make informed decisions affecting my life. I hope I can inspire others to do the same—to set their sights, chart their courses, and realize their goals. Through that process, I hope they will realize their options and, more important, that we are all truly connected and individually we *can* make a difference in the lives of others.

Eat Ice Cream for Breakfast

You've got breast cancer."

I remember the day and the tears that fell. The doctor couldn't have been talking to me. Had she picked up the wrong file? Did she have the wrong Colette?

No, it was true—it was me. Those words seared through me like a wild brushfire. A few days before hearing the bad news, I had lunch with a group of girlfriends. When I heard that one in eight women gets breast cancer, I was glad it was me and not one of my friends. It would have been far more painful to see my friends suffer. Kitty likes her hair too much. Martha likes her boobs too much. P.J. hates bad sunburn. And the list went on.

I thought only old people got cancer. I thought it only happened to the guy at the post office or the lady who lived in Texas who once knew your uncle. I didn't know until that day that it could actually happen to me. How does it happen? Where does it come from? And how do I send it back?

Who cares? I decided I wasn't going to have anything to do with it. All I had to do was look at my two little boys and the answer was clear—I had to fight. It was that simple. They were so young. Four-year-old Bazil and two-year-old Cecil were too young to understand what was about to happen.

I decided to serve ice cream for breakfast. As Bazil and I ate Rocky Road and Cecil ate Mint Chip, I kept the explanation simple. I told the boys I was going to have surgery and some strong medicine and that I would lose all of my hair. Bazil translated for his baby brother. "Mommy's boobies are sick and the doctor is going to take them off so the rest of Mommy won't get sick," he said.

I had a double mastectomy followed by the "hair today, gone tomorrow" chemotherapy and six weeks of radiation. Because of the large amount of scar tissue created by the radiation, I then found out I was not a candidate for reconstruction. I still remember telling Louise, my oncology nurse, that I had always wanted bigger boobs and curly hair. I didn't get either but now realize that what I got was worth far more.

Cancer can't get to my heart or my soul.

It is the part of me that you can't see that is so special. It is on the inside, my heart and my soul. Cancer can't get to my heart or my soul. I remain strong and positive. Even though I'm a hairdresser and in the "beauty business," I have always believed that true beauty is more than just skin deep.

Cancer has been far more painful for the people around me: my family, my friends, my coworkers, and even my doctors. Breast cancer doesn't hurt. It is silent and it changes the lives of everyone who is affected by it.

My cancer has changed other people's lives to the point where I have started to believe that things really do happen for a reason. I was the chosen one. What happened to me was a gift, of sorts. People started telling me it was a wake-up call. They started to live their lives in an unaffected way. The fancy cars, the diamond rings, and the second homes somehow seemed irrelevant. Material things don't count in the end. Nor do they count in the big picture. People started realizing this and it made me so happy!

Part of my saving grace was Peggy, a longtime client and friend and a breast cancer survivor herself. She was always off skiing or white-water rafting. She went on with her life as though nothing had changed. And so did Jackie. She was my other hero. Jackie was a breast cancer survivor, too, and was always flying around judging dog shows and telling tales. These gals gave me hope.

Then there was Joanne, who was near my age, recently diagnosed with cancer and in desperate need of a wig. We worked together and created one that looked just like her hair, if not a bit better.

Two years after my surgery, the doctors recommended that I have a radical hysterectomy to stop the production of hormones because the medicine I was taking wasn't performing as well as they had hoped. No big deal. I was 42 and had had both of my beautiful boys by C-section, so I asked if they could do the surgery with an epidural. I was awake, chatting with my doctor and the nurses. The only difference is they don't hand you a baby at the end.

Just a few months ago, I found another lump on my chest. It seems as if breast cancer isn't picky about springing the news on you. I was leaving in four days with the boys for a vacation to the south of France when I got the news. My doctor said, "Are you sure you want the results before you go?"

"Yes," I said, "because I'm either going to have peace of mind or I'm going to buy 10 pairs of shoes in Paris."

Two days later she called and said, "Buy the shoes."

I did just that: Burberry, Chanel, and Prada. The boys and I had a blast. We stayed in Cannes and went to the beach every day followed by our afternoon merry-go-round ride. We ate too much, slept in every day, and stayed up as late as we could every night. For two little guys, that was a big deal! We lived each day like tomorrow might not arrive.

Two weeks ago, I had the lump removed. The margins were clear and I'm back to cutting hair and telling stories. The best advice I can give anyone, breast cancer or not, is to live your life. After all, isn't that what we're supposed to do?

Karen J. Shirey, Ph.D.

A Woman's Best Friends

A bullhorn-sounding school bell blasts—again—and then a final peel.

Silence.

The horn comes again.

It's another day in my life as a high school counselor. The students who parade in and out of my office don't notice anything different. I guess for all outward appearances, I look the same, but under all my clothes lies a secret few people know.

I have no breasts.

* * *

Today, it's no secret. I want everyone to know. I celebrate all the anniversaries (cancer surgery dates, a new yearly prosthesis, when I returned to work), and I want everyone to celebrate with me. So much has happened in my life; every day is a new day.

In the fall of 1988, divorce was the dreaded word and not cancer. Earlier in the day, I'd come home from the courthouse. My divorce was final. My second marriage was over, and I was not yet 40 years old. While I wasn't worried for myself financially, I did feel like a failure. I'd failed in love, not once, but twice. How did it happen? How could it happen to me? I wondered how my professional life could be so good and my personal life such a mess. I had to face facts—my life wasn't what I expected it to be.

"It's good that both of my ex-husbands are still my friends," I said to comfort myself. As I sat on the couch, lovingly stroking the heads of my two buff-colored cocker spaniels, Winchester and Remington, who looked at me with unconditional love, I realized I was starting over, again.

As the months slipped by and the winter holidays were approaching, I was determined not to sit home and mope. I'd already decided to chaperone the high school's winter dance and participate in homecoming week.

The first week of December, I reported as customary for my annual physical. Nothing unusual to report, but my doctor needed to review the results of the mammogram and would call if anything suspicious showed up.

I'll never forget the date, December 24, 1988. My parents and I were sitting down to Christmas Eve dinner when the phone rang. "I'm sorry to call you on Christmas Eve, with bad news," the doctor said, "but I thought it was important for you to know that we found a tumor in your right breast."

Two days later, the biopsy was performed. The report from the pathologists came back positive for cancer. It was noninvasive, meaning it hadn't spread—a lump in the milk duct, easy to remove. The prognosis and possibility for cure were good. But visions of red, scraggly scars that crisscrossed my mother's chest from her cancer surgery back in the early 1960s reminded me of her legacy.

"What if it was your wife, what would you do?" I asked my doctor.

"Be progressive and aggressive," was his answer.

Searching the Web, I e-mailed a couple of veterinarians and oncologists who once worked with my first husband, Dr. Jim Shirey. Days later, I barely controlled my voice when I heard Jim say, "Hello," on the other end of the phone. He called because someone had sent him a copy of my e-mail. We hadn't spoken for two years, and here he was offering innovative options and concern for my health. His soft, smooth voice calmed my ragged nerves. His genuine concern made me wonder why I hadn't made more of an effort to stay in touch, but I remembered we both were married at the time. We talked for over an hour. He was divorced again and, like me, he didn't have any children. It was as if we'd never been apart. Just before we ended the call, he told me that he'd be there for me.

When I awoke from the surgery, I knew my breast was gone. My fingertips explored the thick padding over the wound. I'd lost a body part, but I had lived through it. I opened my eyes, determined to face another day. Imagine my surprise when I saw Jim sitting with my parents by the bed. I never expected him to fly back from his conference just to be here with me, but that's exactly what he did.

Jim's presence and my mother's success at beating her breast cancer fueled my confidence and eased my worries. I won't deny that at first it felt like I'd been given a death sentence. I faced my mortality, felt the pain, and grieved the loss. But the early diagnosis was a chance to live.

Without regret, I chose not to have reconstructive surgery. I didn't want to worry about mammograms or the possibility that the cancer could come back and hide behind the implants. If the cancer should return, I wanted to find it and get rid of it immediately. Besides, it was my body and it was my decision to make. If a man with whom I became romantic didn't like that I didn't have a breast, then I would end the relationship. No man was deciding my future.

It turned out that Jim and I started dating again, and he became an important part of my recovery. Jim didn't pity me. I wouldn't stand for it. I'd had cancer. It was gone, and now I was getting on with life. And our life together was better. We were starting over. Our new maturity brought a new beginning. I learned that just because my breast was gone love wasn't unromantic. It's all about acceptance, no matter what condition you're in. We value being alive and together. By June, we remarried. I got my high school sweetheart and my best friend back.

> *I LEARNED THAT JUST because my breast was gone love wasn't unromantic. It's all about acceptance, no matter what condition you're in.*

But my new life looked far different on me. My chest was lopsided with a nasty red scar where my old boob had been for so many years. I tried stuffing my bra with socks, nylons, or toilet paper. Suddenly, my preadolescent tricks brought a whole new meaning to turning 40.

When I went back to school, the students had no idea there was anything different. But many of my colleagues, particularly the men, didn't know where or how to look at me. Covertly, they'd sneak a peek at my breasts, instead of keeping eye contact, trying to determine the fake breast. Not missing a beat, I'd tell them, "It's the right one." Many times I was tempted to keep my eyes on their crotch while talking to them, but decided my bluntness would only embarrass and probably alienate them. We all needed to adjust, and I realized I was the one who would have to set the standard.

The following annual physical revealed cancer in the other breast. The doctors had denied my earlier request to have the other breast removed. But this time was easier. I challenged myself to recover faster, setting a goal of returning to work earlier than the last experience, hoping to set a record.

Now at least I wasn't lopsided. But I had a while before I could use my prosthesis, so I turned back to the old reliable socks. It's funny—small-breasted women will identify with me when I say how hard it is to achieve that full-breasted look when you have no breasts at all. Stuffing socks or hosiery inside my bra was only part of the problem. How do you keep the bra from moving up and down? One minute it's in place, and the next it's moved up under my armpits. Somehow, I had to anchor my bra in place. Taking a shoelace, I tied it to my bra, and safety-pinned the shoelace to my underpants. Great! But what do I do when I have to use the toilet? No one tells you about these things. When the shoelace wouldn't work, I tried putting BBs, those tiny lead balls used in BB guns, in the bra cup, weighing it down. But sooner or later, the BBs fell through the cracks, bouncing on the ground, making the simple act of walking difficult. Imagine this picture—my arms hanging down, pressed tightly against my sides, trying to keep my bra from riding up, while I gingerly maneuver the BBs on the ground. It's not a pretty sight!

Technology has kept up, making fake appliances that look and feel real. But one option I never had when I had my own breasts was the option of going without a bra. Ah, what a feeling of freedom! But now it's freedom to choose wearing boobs or going boobless, and I can change the size of my breasts, too. I can just stick them on and go. I use what makes me feel comfortable.

Before I married Jim, I guess I could say that I had two other male friends, Winchester and Remington. They were family, the children I would never have. When I had surgery and came home from the hospital, those two cockers stayed with me. Winchester would stretch out on the couch along my thigh, his feet in the air, softly snoring, while Remington sat curled up in a tight ball on my lap. Sooner or later, Remington would stretch out across my lap, his head hanging over one side and his back legs hanging over the other side, a big 30-pound lump of curly golden fur. Escape from the couch was rare; whenever it became necessary, those two guys were never far behind.

I told them Mommy was sick and had to take things easy. A moment later, Winchester tapped my hand with his paw. I reached over to pet him behind the ears, but he started licking my hand before I reached him. Remington just looked at me with his droopy chocolate-brown eyes before settling back against the cushions. It was all right with them if we took life slower.

The dogs loved to play, particularly with plastic toys. One way or another they managed to bury everything, including their nylon bone. Once, when I was digging up the garden to plant a few vegetables, I found the missing garage-door opener.

Right after I'd had my second surgery, we were hosting a small party. I wanted to see my friends and colleagues in private. I was dressing when everyone started arriving. Winchester and Remington were playing with an old toy, a white sock that Jim had stuffed with a tennis ball. I heard some yipping and low growling, not uncommon for those two. I heard their scuffling feet sliding across the floor as I came out of the bathroom, slipping a blouse over my head. Out of the corner of my eye, I caught sight of them swiping their toy with their paws, scooting it across the hardwood floor. I settled the blouse before reaching for the gray slacks on the bed. The beige toy lay between them as they panted, momentarily out of breath.

Then it dawned on me. B-e-i-g-e. "Oh, no," I thought, dropping the pants and staring at what I suspected—the dogs' toy was my prosthesis. "Remington, come here and bring your toy," I ordered. Remington picked up the pliable lump with teeth marks along the casing. Then Winchester tried to take it out of his mouth.

"Come here, and bring your toy to Mommy." I snapped my fingers, moving quietly toward the dogs. They sidestepped my outreached hand and loped away, heading for the bedroom door. "Remington, come here." I quickened my pace and followed him. Winchester barged in between us, and the two tugged and pulled on the boob. They started downstairs, but because I was half dressed and we had company downstairs, I couldn't follow. I raced back to the bedroom, pulled on my pants as fast as I could, and ran down the stairs in time to see Remington prance through the house, his mouth filled with my prosthesis, on his way to the backyard.

"Grab him, Jim," I yelled.

"Sorry, honey, they're too quick," Jim responded. "Besides, it's just their burgers."

One of our guests, who was in the backyard with the dogs, reported, "You have to see this. Remington dropped his toy and Winchester picked it up. They were playing tug-of-war, and now they're busy digging a hole."

We stepped outside. Both furry mutts were busy letting dirt fly under the tree as they yipped and yelped, their paws working furiously in the dirt. A moment later, they looked up, dark mud stuck to their noses. Turning around, they began covering their treasure.

"It's not their burgers," I said to Jim. "They're trying to bury my prosthesis."

At that point, I realized there was nothing I could do. So I started laughing. It took me a few moments before I could say anything. "I have to tell you all something . . . that toy, well, it wasn't a toy." I stopped, holding everyone's attention. "What they buried was my prosthesis." Blank stares returned my gaze. "You know . . . my fake boobs." I waited, while the two cockers continued burying their prize. "It's all right," I chuckled. It took a moment before everyone realized what was happening and they joined in the laughter.

"I guess I won't be wearing those anymore," I paused. "Two hundred fifty dollars of soft rubber buried in our backyard, a real family treasure."

> *Nothing was unmanageable with a positive attitude.*

As embarrassing as their foray was, I realized that life held many of those moments, no more embarrassing with or without disabilities. Nothing was unbearable with the help of my best friends: Jim, Remington, and Winchester. Nothing was unmanageable with a positive attitude.

Olivia's Lessons

W hen I asked the mother of another child in my daughter's preschool class what she told her daughter when she was diagnosed with breast cancer, she said, "I didn't tell her anything more than I have a boo-boo that needs help from a doctor and that I'll be all right."

I thought for a three-year-old, that was sufficient, but for Olivia, my precocious five-year-old, it would not be enough of an explanation to satisfy her curious mind.

How and what I told her evolved over the process of the diagnosis, surgery, and treatments. I knew that it was not the words as much as how I said them that would really make the difference.

We started with the word "boo-boo" while I was going through the biopsy period. The afternoon I found out it was cancer, I went into the backyard and cried. There is a wooded valley behind our home, and I stood in the middle of the trees and sobbed. Olivia was inside with our afternoon sitter,

Jamie. I thought I would fall apart if the biopsy came back as cancer. But I didn't. After letting it all out, I felt a deep sense of calm. I knew I had to deal with the cancer no matter how upset it made me, and I had to tell Olivia what had happened right away, while I was relatively calm.

"If I'm okay when I tell her, she'll be okay," I told myself. So I went back inside and sat on the couch in the den with Jamie on one side and Olivia on the other. I put my arm around my daughter's shoulders and said, "Olivia, I'm sorry I was crying a few minutes ago, but I got some news that made me feel sad and afraid. Remember how I told you the doctor was checking the boo-boo?" I inquired. "Well, the doctor found out that it is a very bad boo-boo and I have to have some surgery to remove it."

Her big blue eyes peered at me, reflecting fear, concern, and love. "Are they going to cut off your breast, Mommy?" she asked.

"No, honey, just some tissue inside it," I responded, stroking her long dark brown hair.

Then she asked a question she would ask for months after that. "Mommy, what started all this?" she wanted to know.

"No one knows for certain, but many people are trying to find that answer," I told her. "Just because this happened to Mommy doesn't mean this will happen to you. Remember, *you* grew in Melissa's body instead of mine. I'm going to need lots of hugs, Olivia, okay?"

One great piece of advice I received was from Meredith Cooper, a counselor who works with families and children. She told me to remember that children are very visual and to be careful about how much I showed her. The memory of what she would see could be very frightening and disturbing.

So I only let her view things she asked to see and only after a little preparation of what it was going to look like. For example, when Olivia asked to see the surgery place, I told her that it was a little swollen and kind of bruised and before I would let her see it, it would have to heal a bit. Also, I let her touch anything that she wanted to touch, which included stitches and incision sites.

When we found out that I was going to have to go through chemotherapy, I told Olivia, "The doctors are going to give me medicine that will destroy the boo-boo cancer cells and it will be very strong. I might feel very sick and my hair will fall out, but it will grow back." Then I asked her, "Would you like me to wear a wig or just hats or scarves when I don't have any hair?"

She preferred that I wear a wig, and that was fine with me. Every day, Olivia would check my bald head like a farmer checking his garden. I was so happy for her on the day she could say, "Mommy, I see some tiny hairs; it's growing back!"

Seeing me look more like myself was reassuring to her. What also helped was a journal she kept in her Montessori kindergarten classroom. Each child writes in a journal as part of the morning routine. Olivia's teacher told me that Olivia eagerly wrote in the journal and that she was surprised to see what Olivia had written. When her teacher showed the journal to me, it was heartbreaking and strangely freeing at the same time.

As I opened the green paper-covered journal, I found the words she had written on half-sized sheets of white lined paper: "My mom is sick and I am sad . . . she still goes to chemotherapy."

Her words and sweet, inexperienced handwriting brought tears to my eyes. I wanted so much to protect her from pain. I continued reading and saw the next entry: "My mom is feeling better today and I am glad. My mom has a bald head but my mom has a little bit of hair. Yesterday my mom did a lot of stuff. I am glad." And then, the next entry: "My mom played with me and I am glad she did. My mom loves me."

It was freeing for me because Olivia had found a constructive way to deal with my illness and its effects on her and on our family. She had found a place to express her feelings and a place of comfort within

She had found a place to express her feelings and a place of comfort within herself. She was coping.

herself. She was coping. The journal helped Olivia take her feelings from the inside and put them on paper, which freed her to move forward into her school environment and her own work. Olivia was very private about her journal. We looked at it together when she brought it home from school, and then she wanted me to put it away.

One day after my last chemotherapy treatment, I was lying in bed and she came in and said, "Mom, just get up! Get out of that bed. Get up!"

She was mad, and although I couldn't quite get up and play yet, I was so glad that she was not protecting me from her feelings. She needed me and believed I should just get over it. She taught me a great deal about honesty and getting on with things. Olivia also taught me that having a purpose is a huge part of healing and survival.

So many times, people keep things from children until later in the process. I believe that kids, like adults, need and deserve the time to process information and their feelings. And if we adults really listen to what they're thinking and feeling, we can learn some valuable lessons from them.

Experimenting with Life

After I underwent surgery, chemotherapy, and radiation therapy for breast cancer, it only seemed natural for me to participate in some studies related to breast cancer. As an employee at the Detroit Medical Center for more than 20 years, I was to raise money for cancer research programs there as part of my job.

I've seen how much has been gained from people who have been quiet heroes, giving their time to participate in cancer studies so that new drugs can be developed, the value of nutrition can be determined, and most important, many forms of cancer will no longer be associated with the term "death sentence." Literally millions of people are alive today, enjoying fulfilling healthy lives after cancer treatment.

I'll never forget a man I talked with about 15 years ago who was diagnosed with cancer in his 30s. He was given only a 5 percent chance of beating his disease. With two daughters to raise, he was determined to live. He's still alive today, thanks to new treatments developed at that time.

Now it was my chance to participate and add my contribution to the fight against breast cancer.

One day as I sat at my office desk reading the daily electronic news for employees on my computer screen, my eyes locked on a headline announcing a walking study. The Wayne State University School of Nursing was conducting the study. Its goal was to determine how increased exercise through a weekly walking program would affect the body, stamina, and emotions of women who had breast cancer.

So three times during the year of the study, on my lunch hour, I would exchange my work pumps for a pair of white walking shoes and, wearing my business suit, I would head to a local health club, where I met a researcher. I felt a little out of place with all those exercisers in their gym suits and workout sweats, but I didn't have time to change and really didn't need to anyway.

Before each walking session, I spent half an hour filling out three detailed questionnaires about how I felt emotionally and physically. Then, with a yellow cloth tape measure, the researcher took hip, thigh, and calf measurements in a private room. We went up the stairs to the oval track, and she stood on the sidelines with a stopwatch and timed each lap as I walked as fast as I could 13 times around the oval orange- and brown-carpeted three-lane track for a total of 1 mile. The first session took me over 15 minutes to complete that mile, my heart pounding and breathing labored. It was hard because I never had been serious about exercise and had gradually put on more than 40 pounds over my ideal weight. The study required a minimum of walking on my own 30 to 45 minutes three times a week. During bad weather, I would walk in the parking deck at work. The inclines of the parking levels gave me an extra good workout. As time went by, my pace quickened and my stamina improved, and by the third and final meeting with the researcher, I shaved minutes off that mile with normal breathing and a smile on my face.

The results haven't been tabulated yet, but I know that, in my case, it worked to improve my energy level and my overall feeling of well-being. Now my goal is to walk at least an hour a day five or six days a week.

I have also lost weight thanks to another study I did concurrently with the walking study. The 24-month diet study was to determine if weight loss can lessen the chance of breast cancer recurrence. I had to write a record of everything I ate, how long I exercised, and what type of workout I did, as well as undergoing periodic body composition measurements and taking blood samples. I spoke weekly with the study nutritionist and attended local Weight Watchers meetings faithfully. I'm proud to say I reached my weight loss goal in nine months. I feel terrific and look pretty good, too!

> *I* KNOW THAT, IN *my case, walking worked to improve my energy level and my overall feeling of well-being.*

I never felt like a "guinea pig" during these studies. The researchers were there to help me, and as a result, I was filling their need to study breast cancer survivors.

At times, having breast cancer made me feel very alone and frightened, but participating in these studies has assured me that my experience will help others, and that makes me feel very good. I hope others will become part of important research so that more of us can beat breast cancer.

Penny Sinisi

Knowledge Is Power

I almost canceled my yearly mammogram. It just wasn't a convenient time. A voice inside told me not to, because, you see, I knew that one day I would get breast cancer. My mother had had it and almost daily she had worried aloud about whether it had come back or, for example, if her headache had meant that cancer was now imbedded in her brain.

Looking back at my mother's obsession with her cancer, I remember how hard it was for me when I was 13 years old. Today I don't know whether to be angry about it or grateful for it. Maybe it's both. I am angry because I wanted my mother to get on with her life. I'm grateful because the knowledge of her diagnosis made me more aware that I could get breast cancer.

That's exactly what happened when I was 47 years old and teaching fifth grade in Kansas City. I was in the teachers' lounge having my usual 25-minute lunch before afternoon classes began. "There is a phone call for Ms. Sinisi," I heard over the intercom.

When I picked up the phone, I heard my doctor's nurse tell me, "Something isn't right with your mammogram, and we have already scheduled a sonogram for you."

I slowly shuffled back to the table where my sandwich waited on top of clear plastic wrap. I sat in a daze and tried to eat my lunch and hide the fear, but I couldn't. The tears started to flow and I lost my appetite.

I HAVE ALWAYS TOLD my students that education is power, and now that lesson rang true for me.

Another teacher saw me cry and tried to reassure me. "It doesn't mean you have cancer," she said. My mother's brainwashing convinced me that I did.

The surgeon confirmed my suspicions when I awoke from the biopsy. "You have a 1.5-centimeter tumor in your right breast," he said.

I took a practical approach and decided not to spend my time worrying about the future, but rather, taking care of business.

Luckily, a good friend was not teaching at the time because she was on maternity leave. We teamed up to find out as much as we could about breast cancer and the surgical options. Pam was also the daughter of a breast cancer survivor, and when I expressed gratitude for her help, she responded, "You'll probably have to do this for me someday; I'm just doing it first."

I have always told my students that education is power, and now that lesson rang true for me. Pam and I went to the newest and biggest bookstore in town and hungrily searched for books about breast cancer. We looked for the women's health section, and I found several volumes to buy. I settled on clinical books with big words and horrid pictures and chapters with headings like "When All Treatments Have Failed." I decided to buy the books, not borrow them, because I wanted to be able to write notes in the margins. I also needed the books to take into the surgeon's office in an effort to let him know he was dealing with a well-informed person.

When I was diagnosed eight years ago, the majority of women just went along with what the doctors told them, but I didn't know my surgeon and I wasn't going to let him tell me what to do before I knew all the options. Lumpectomies with subsequent radiation were relatively new, at least here in the Middle West.

Pam's and my arms were filled with books about breast cancer when we arrived at the surgeon's office. I was hoping to intimidate him with my knowledge, because I had a feeling that he would want to perform a mastectomy. "We'll be able to schedule the mastectomy within 10 days," he said, as if that were the only possible surgical solution.

With a great deal of trepidation at first and then with a voice steadily gaining strength, I told the surgeon, "I'm single, in my mid-40s, and someday I'd like to have a date, maybe even a significant relationship. Having only one breast would [at least to my way of thinking at the time] make that more difficult."

When I followed up my monologue with a question about whether I'd be a good candidate for a lumpectomy, the surgeon tilted his head to one side, noticed the books, and decided that the less invasive procedure might work after all. We both agreed that if my lymph nodes were clear and all indicators were positive, I would follow up my surgery with only radiation, no chemotherapy. And that's what happened.

Those breast cancer books no longer sit idly on my bookshelves. I have loaned them to other women who have been diagnosed and who want to make educated decisions about their future.

Nancy Carstedt

So Much to Live For

Battling breast cancer changed me from desperately wanting to die to desperately wanting to live.

When I was dealing with depression and alcoholism about 20 years ago, dying seemed like it would have been a welcomed relief. Things were so bad that twice I tried to kill myself.

My depression started after my mother died, and it grew worse when my husband of 20 years left our marriage and our three children, and married a good friend.

It was hard on all of us. My son, a freshman in high school at the time, attempted suicide and failed. In a flash, my once independent son became a quadriplegic and I, now a single mother of three, was in charge of his demanding, around-the-clock caretaking.

Before facing each day, I'd have a drink of white wine for breakfast and another wine glass full for snacks and other meals throughout the day. "If only I could die," I thought, "then I wouldn't feel all of the pain inside of me."

Within 18 months, I became a fall-down drunk and went into the hospital for treatment. After becoming sober, the depression was unmasked and I sank so low that I spent 15 months in a psychiatric hospital.

It took five years before I was depression- and alcohol-free and was able to build a beautiful life for myself.

Then, *boom!* My life changed again when, in January of 2000, I went for my annual mammogram, and cancer was found in my left breast and in my lymph nodes. I underwent a lumpectomy and axillary dissection, followed by six months of chemotherapy and eight weeks of radiation and a year of weekly intravenous herceptin treatments. Throughout them, I asked God not to let me die. I had so much to live for!

Over the years, I have seen my two daughters marry, and I have been blessed to have four grandchildren. I have also been rewarded by my work as executive director of the Chicago Children's Choir, involving 3,000 children between the ages of 8 and 18, most of whom come from low-income, minority homes.

> *THE BREAST CANCER diagnosis became a wake-up call. It made me realize that I wanted to experience my life, not lose it.*

Instead of throwing me into a depression or to alcohol, the breast cancer diagnosis became a wake-up call. It made me realize that I wanted to experience my life, not lose it. I followed the doctor's suggestions and am cancer-free.

I smile when I look back at the time my daughters surprised me during one of my chemotherapy treatments. When I came home exhausted and opened the front door, I heard music playing and saw my three grandsons, aged two, four, and six, wearing brightly colored bathing trunks and straw sombreros. In the family room, there was 100 pounds of sand. My family was going to create a Mexican beach for me because I had to cancel a trip to Mexico to make time for chemotherapy. Our being able to laugh and cry together made a huge difference in my recovery.

It was also helpful to be surrounded by so many sweet and loving children at work. Some days, kids would come into my office and ask, "Need a hug today?" Their little arms around my neck and body brought such a sense of hope for the future.

The year following chemotherapy, I took each of my adult children on a trip that reflected their interests. My son and I traveled to Lake Tahoe to see comedian George Carlin. My older daughter and her family went with me to Disney World in Florida, and my younger daughter and I made that long-awaited trip to Mexico.

Time has always been a precious commodity, but sometimes it takes a life-threatening illness to make us appreciate it. Now I make time each week to spend a day with my grandsons, enjoying the simple pleasures of being there to see them grow.

Thank goodness my prayers were answered so that I could live to see my oldest daughter marry and bless my life with four wonderful grandsons, and now I am being blessed again with the marriage of my youngest daughter.

Never Give Up

I had spent five long nights in the hospital. My time was filled with hours and hours of tests—scans, and blood work, pokings and proddings, interns and specialists, phone calls and visitors, good wishes and my own fear. My doctor phoned and said he would give me some answers at 10:00 A.M. He told me to make sure my husband was there. The waiting was over. The diagnosis was in.

I watched the doctor carefully as he sat on my bed. I caught his eye, but he looked away. Then I heard the words. I shook my head. "Oh, really," was all I could say as I fought back the tears. I did not know what the doctor's words really meant. The diagnosis echoed in my head even though I did not understand the implications. The words almost didn't matter. I knew I was sick. I knew I was tired. I knew I wanted to go home to my 10-year-old son. But even then, at the start of my journey, I sensed that life as I had known it and lived it and wanted to live it was over. I felt alone with my weighty diagnosis. Stage 4 breast cancer. The cancer had already spread from my right breast to both of my lungs.

Now, after more than two years of living with it, I can say I understand what metastatic breast cancer is. It is a full-time endeavor. I have noticed that when women are treated for early stage breast cancer, they wonder how they will ever get over the experience and get back to their lives. When diagnosed with late stage cancer, you wonder how you will make a new life incorporating the experience. When I am not being treated or tested (or waiting for results), I am educating myself about my disease. I have learned about the biology of cancer. I can now draw lovely pictures of a cell and define angiogenesis. I can name the clinical trials in my region. I have read books, scientific and lay. I know cancer treatment is political—I can name the congresspeople who support breast cancer funding legislation. I understand how a plethora of drugs work.

You can't fight cancer with knowledge alone. It takes a spiritual healing as well.

But you can't fight cancer with knowledge alone. It takes a spiritual healing as well. When I started to feel physically better (being on weekly chemo for a year) after surgery to re-inflate my collapsed lung, I looked for something to help heal my spirit. I was told my disease was not curable, but I felt that metastatic cancer is more than a physical disease. While the body must fight for its life against a systemic enemy (against incredible odds), for me the most difficult battle has been the mental and spiritual. While I have intellectually tried to come to terms with my diagnosis, I realized it might be impossible for me to ever understand. I needed to find a combination of something physical to help my body heal and something that would help my mind and my spirit.

Many things and people have kept me going. One of them is Mr. Gu, a man who teaches a special, healing form of exercise. When I first went to Mr. Gu's class, the exercises seemed very hard to me—my energy level was low and it was difficult for me to do them correctly. He assigned a woman to help me, to push me, to make sure I did the exercises frequently and correctly. That was 10 months ago. I now do some form of his exercises each day, and I see him once a week. I feel great. I have a lot more energy, and I am able to keep up in class. My last CT scan showed no evidence of disease. This is my second clean CT scan. I feel that doing Mr. Gu's exercises (and speaking with Mr. Gu) has put me on the path of recovery. He has a wonderful energy, and he generously shares it with his students.

The exercises themselves are unlike any other I've ever heard of. Mr. Gu has developed a total system to enhance your energy and "massage" your vital organs. The exercises themselves are a unique combination of massage, aerobics, yoga, and reflexology designed to make you feel better, energized, and healthier. And I am energized by what I have learned from Mr. Gu.

Living with cancer, I have learned that I must find ways to take care of my body and my soul. The greatest lesson may be that the spirit is impervious to the diagnosis. It is this realization that lets me fight when I know there is currently no cure for stage 4 disease. Statistically, the odds are not in my favor. I have buried many friends and fear there will be many more funerals for me to attend in the future. But I believe I am more than my diagnosis. I believe (odd as it may sound) that I am healed, even though my cancer can never be cured. Because I am healed, I feel up to the task of difficult fights: I had a tough battle to get out of the hospital (I was there for almost a month). But with stage 4 breast cancer, there are no easy answers, no pretty pictures, and no looking back with fondness. Only a fight for your life. Nothing is guaranteed or certain. My plan is to battle for a long time. To that end, I will continue with Mr. Gu and my exercises. That is my plan. The only thing I know for sure is that I will die fighting.

Jane R. Handwerk

The Bridge Is There

I was celebrating my first year of remission from breast cancer in early October 1999. It was almost a year to the day as I walked with a group of very special friends across the Walnut Street Bridge in Harrisburg, Pennsylvania, during the city's first American Cancer Society's Making Strides Against Breast Cancer Walk. We ranged in age from the early 30s to 81, and we wore white T-shirts emblazoned with large navy and bright pink letters advertising our exercise group's name, The Fitness Fanatics. As we enthusiastically walked over the old iron-trussed, arched bridge, our footsteps were echoed by a sea of approximately 500 people who joined us in this historic walk.

As this lively, upbeat assemblage of color zigzagged down the ramp from the old iron river span, then looped under the bridge along the shore pathway, I was reminded of the children's game in which a continuous line of brightly colored marbles rolled down a winding track. From the top to the bottom, the marbles would circle around and around (*clickety clack, clickety clack*) until finally coming to a rest at the end. Just like the walkers, there was a special rhythm and enthusiasm because of the shared common cause.

Breast cancer statistics are chilling, as chilling as the rapid and frigid Susquehanna River flowing beneath the bridge we were walking over that day. But more and more of us who have had breast cancer are making it across the bridge from diagnosis of fear and death to the other side where life, health, and survivorship reside.

I was 56 when breast cancer was diagnosed. Being a lifelong optimist, I had not been overly concerned about the lump that I had found in my right breast during a monthly breast self-exam.

Once the diagnosis was made, my emotions caught up with me and I cried. The shock and surprise had moved on to fear. I had cancer! Cancer? Other people got cancer, not me. Although I've always known I was as much a candidate as anyone else in the world, I had always thought that I might be one of the lucky ones, one who did not get cancer.

Now, as I was walking with my friends above those cold-rushing waters, I knew I truly was one of the lucky ones because I have survived. I look back at the lumpectomy, the radiation therapy, and the four going on five years of taking tamoxifen, and I feel blessed. I did not need chemotherapy. I did not lose a breast or my hair or my lunch on any day. Instead of being unwilling to accept having the disease, I told myself, "You have breast cancer. You must fight it and go on with your life."

I thank God every day for allowing me to be a cancer survivor and to experience a sunrise and a sunset. I am proud to have joined an elite group of women who have gone through hell to fight for life.

The year prior to my diagnosis and the years that have followed the first walk have been exceptional when I consider the advances made in breast cancer therapy, including the new drugs, treatments, and in-depth education that are available. All of this progress was unknown to me the day my surgeon told me that I had breast cancer.

For as long as I live, I have vowed to continue to celebrate life by participating in this walk. Each year that I do, I walk not only for myself, but for all the women and men who have faced and will have to deal with the trauma of being told they have breast cancer.

> *I* TOLD MYSELF, *"You have breast cancer. You must fight it and go on with your life."*

When I look back at how breast cancer came into my life, I realize that my story is not about the day I was diagnosed, or the lumpectomy, or those six weeks of early morning radiation treatments. My story is about triumph. It is about crossing a bridge to the side of strength and remission from breast cancer. It's about being able to tell my story. Each year as I walk across that bridge with a group that has grown to more than 4,000 walkers, the symbolism of the bridge does not escape me. By participating, I want to help others find strength and courage and a new perspective on life on the other side of the bridge. It's there. The challenge is for us to take the steps to reach it.

Moments

W ill my life ever really be the same? Could I actually die, even though they caught it early? Will my new employers still want me to take the job? Was I going to be unemployed *and* endure breast cancer? Being single and having no other steady source of income, I found this to be a very frightening thought.

Those thoughts kept racing through my mind in the moments after learning a biopsy determined the white spots that appeared on my right breast during a routine mammogram were precancerous. What did they mean by precancerous? Does that mean I just barely missed the bullet? "It means you have an area of abnormal cells that have not yet begun to destroy good cells," my primary doctor told me. "You're lucky they caught it at this stage. You will probably need a lumpectomy and some low-grade radiation, that's it." Somehow I didn't feel all that lucky. Apparently I wasn't part of the vast majority of biopsies that come back free and clear.

I suppose there's no convenient time for breast cancer to be diagnosed, but I couldn't imagine a worse moment in my life to get the news. I had just quit my job and had accepted another position as an office manager for an insurance brokerage firm. I had been looking for a position just like this for a very long time. It was perfect! I was supposed to attend the wedding of one of my new employers just a few days after my diagnosis and then start work shortly thereafter. But I could not think about any of this now. The following week, I was scheduled for my first appointment with a surgeon and I wanted to be well informed.

Determined I was going to handle this just fine and with a long list of questions in hand regarding lumpectomies and the effects of radiation, I felt prepared for the next step. As I sat nervously in my hospital gown, one of the doctors sat down on a small stool in front of me. The look on his face warned me that the next thing out of his mouth was not going to be good. "The type of cancer you have has a very high chance of recurrence if treated with a lumpectomy," he said. "Also this approach would be cosmetically undesirable because the affected area is too big. I'm sorry to say we will have to take the whole thing."

None of my research prepared me for this. "How high is the risk of recurrence if we do the lumpectomy?" I asked. "And how did it get so big in the year since my last clear mammogram?"

"The chances of recurrence are 20 to 50 percent, and we suspect it was already there a year ago, but as yet undetectable," he replied.

In the midst of my shock, I managed to ask one last question. "Does this put the left side at equal risk?"

"Yes," was all he said. That pretty much said it all. By late the next day, I had decided to have a double mastectomy with reconstruction.

The next several days were a blur of phone calls, crying spells, and late nights on the Internet. I had to quickly educate myself. Who knew there were so many treatment options?

Next was an office visit with a reconstruction surgeon. This turned into a two-hour ordeal, hearing things I didn't want to hear and ending with a series of pictures I wasn't ready to see, of women in different stages of reconstruction. I left feeling a sense of being violated, and more confused and disillusioned than ever. What made me think it was going to be behind me anytime soon?

Now it was the day before Gayle's wedding. I was just not emotionally equipped to attend what would be a full day of happy events after going through the worst week of my life. What was I going to do? I decided to call Gayle's partner, Laurie, and left a message on her answering machine. Almost as soon as I began talking, I started to cry. "I'm really sorry and don't want to ruin Gayle's wedding," I said while gasping for air, "but I really need to speak with you. I won't be able to start work when I had planned. Can you call me as soon as possible?"

When my phone rang an hour later, it wasn't Laurie but Gayle on the other end. She had picked up Laurie's messages and was calling to see what was wrong. I managed to get out the whole ordeal. She was extremely supportive and then asked, "Do you not want to work for us now?"

"I didn't know if you still wanted me to come," I replied.

Laurie called later and echoed Gayle's sentiments. I felt lucky to have two understanding women as my future employers. It was as if a tremendous weight had been lifted off of my shoulders, enabling me to concentrate on recovering from my upcoming surgery.

This was truly no time to play Wonder Woman. I was hearing about too many women having complications that could have been avoided if they hadn't tried to do too much too soon after surgery. Help and support from family and friends was critical, not to mention vital to my sanity, so I asked my mother and father to fly from New Jersey to California to help take care of me. They readily agreed.

Surgery went through without a hitch. No added surprises to speak of. Emotions were less raw, but still very much present and on the surface. I was healing nicely and anxious to start the reconstruction process. Local support groups were very helpful at this time, supplying everything from rides to appointments to much needed information and emotional support.

Recovering from breast cancer has taught me to have faith in my own strength and resilience—physically, emotionally, in every way.

I write this story eight months after the diagnosis, and I've been working for the insurance brokerage firm ever since. Both Gayle and Laurie, along with many others, have given me the time I've needed to heal and the emotional support on days when my coping and concentration skills haven't been at their best.

Now, as I take time off to undergo the last of my reconstruction, I'm not worried about the future. Whatever happens, and with the help of those around me, I will weather it through.

Right now I am feeling stronger than ever and happy with my life. Recovering from breast cancer has taught me to have faith in my own strength and resilience—physically, emotionally, in every way. I find I am more fully trusting in the process and flow of life, instead of trying to micromanage it. I feel I have more peace now than I had before. This comes from knowing that things do get better, no matter how chaotic, unpredictable, or painful the situation. This may happen gradually and sporadically, but it does happen. It comes from being "more present" with my life, instead of looking back or into the future. This does not mean I have lost sight of my goals or what is most important to me— quite the contrary. Those things have become clearer. The difference now is that I pause and enjoy the journey along the way, not missing one precious moment.

Help Along the Road

A woman, whom I met at a cancer clinic in London, Ontario, when we were both early in treatment, told me she believed that God reached us through the people who came into our lives. Along the road of treatment, with all of its twists and turns, people kept "showing up" for me when I needed them most.

I had a lumpectomy on April 18, 2001. On April 24, my six-year-old daughter was "flying up" from her current level of Sparks in the Girl Scouts club to Brownies. There was a ceremony of sorts at the local elementary school, and she was anxious for me to be there. I could see it in her shining, excited eyes when she asked, "Can you come and watch me, Mom?"

I was still wearing a drainage bag that collected the lymph fluid from the surgery sites. I had already received, before surgery, the astonishing news that I had invasive breast cancer, but the pathology report had since confirmed positive lymph nodes under my arm. I was gearing up for the next long leg of the journey—the chemo—but at this point, I was supposed to heal and recover from the surgery. I was feeling particularly out of sorts that day. I was annoyed by the drainage bag and its long tube. I was constantly besieged by darting, sharp pains through the sites under the arm and through the wound on my breast. I felt that my privacy was disturbed with each arrival of the daily nurse, who would check my wounds and drain the fluid from this bag. And ultimately, I was still reeling in shock that I was in this predicament in the first place. But nonetheless, there was my sweet daughter, and she wanted her mother to go to the Fly Up Ceremony, just like the other mothers were doing.

I did go to my daughter's ceremony, and it was there that I was met by Joan, one of the very many people whom I was to learn would give me the most help for the next 10 months. I knew Joan only in a cursory way, through our children. I was very aware of Joan's eyes watching me as I sat through the ceremony. She did not know of my situation but seemed to sense that I was hurting. Afterward, she came to me, and with her arm around the back of my chair, she said, "I have Level II, Therapeutic Touch, and I would like to help you." Late that evening, Joan came to my home, armed with a blanket, a candle, some lotion, and most important, a deep belief in her ability to help me cope and heal.

I lay upstairs on my bed, covered by Joan's electric wool blanket. At any other time in my life, this would have seemed so odd to me, to be lying there with someone I hardly knew, as she offered me a kind of therapy of which I knew nothing. But learning I had breast cancer had rendered me more in need than I had ever been before, and my own sense of self-preservation told me to accept these friendly offers. Joan explained to me, "I am going to move my hands above your body, but I will not touch you, except for in a few spots, like your ankles. At the end, I will hold your hand. Then you can send me an unspoken request for what you need."

The light fragrance of the candle quickly filled the room, and the light from the candle shone only fleetingly, just enough to create a comfortable atmosphere. I did not know about Therapeutic Touch; I had never even heard the term before, so I was unsure of it, and I chose to keep my eyes closed while Joan slowly moved her hands above my body. At first, I could feel a lot of breeze on my skin, and I thought about Joan having to move her hands that quickly in order to create this fan-like effect. (I later learned that the giver of this kind of touch moves her hands very slowly, almost imperceptibly, and that the energy that she delivers is what I was actually feeling.) I found myself relaxing, letting go and accepting this experience. For the very first time since all of this trauma had invaded my emotional being, I was relaxing, and in that moment, I let out the tears, many of them. They rushed forth out of me in sobs so powerful that I could not hold them back.

My grandmother's image kept coming to my mind. My grandmother was all lilacs and lilies of the valley, whistles and hums, cookies and warm tea. I had missed her deeply since her death many years ago, and since the time when I had first learned of my breast cancer, I had been thinking of her quite often. I had been very close to her, and it was through her that I learned how to nurture and "mother" my own children. Now I needed her to give me strength, of that I was sure. I saw her sweet face, with the soft skin that never seemed to age; I saw her wispy gray hair that I used to pin curl for her; I saw her kind and loving hands, but most of all, I *felt* her presence.

Joan delivered Therapeutic Touch to me for more than 45 minutes that night. Then she touched my hand, as she had prepared me. By this point, I was calm, and in my heart I cried out, "I need my grandmother," although I did not utter a word. Was it some kind of divine intervention, or was it simply the fine intuition of a loving, caring woman that made Joan come to me and hold me tightly with the nurturing arms of my own grandmother pulsing through my memory? Whatever goodness inspired Joan to do it, she held me for a long time, as I wept out in fear, and in sadness and also in hope.

After this, Joan came to my home several times more delivering Therapeutic Touch whenever I asked for it, or whenever she thought I could use it, like before I saw the surgeon again or just before treatment. She never asked for money and assured me that her work was a pleasure for her and a gift to me. Each time, through Joan, I felt the hovering presence of my grandmother's spirit, encouraging me to stay strong, lifting up my heart from its despair. Joan brought me the greatest gift— the awareness that I was not alone and that I would not have to be alone as I embarked on this unplanned, unwanted, but ultimately necessary, journey.

WHAT I HAD NOT expected were the great numbers of virtual strangers who stepped forward, arms open, and guided me along various and difficult parts of the road.

I knew, and even expected, that my closest friends and family would support me through the difficult days of surgery, chemotherapy, and radiation. What I had not expected were the great numbers of virtual strangers who stepped forward, arms open, and guided me along various and difficult parts of the road. These people perceived the time had come for them to be helpful, and hence, they each delivered their special kind of support. Their unsolicited kindness brought back to me my childhood faith—in the presence of God, here among people—a faith I will carry with me for the rest of the way!

Celebrate Life

In January of 2002, I was one of the Seattle-area people chosen to carry the Olympic torch as it made its way across the United States to its final destination at the Olympic games in Salt Lake City, Utah. As someone who is living with stage 4 breast cancer, has survived acute myelogenous leukemia, and has power-walked in seven marathons, I felt honored and up to the challenge.

Wearing our white Olympic uniforms, hats, and gloves, our group of 24 boarded the shuttle bus after posing for a group picture in front of the vehicle. We were half an hour behind schedule, due to trains blocking our route. I had anxiety as I pictured my close-knit group of friends, most of whom I'd met at fund-raising events, waiting outside on one of the coldest nights on record.

When the shuttle bus doors opened, I saw my support group of friends and family with glittered signs that read "Go Tamara" or "You Go Girl!" topped with balloons and confetti streamers. I could feel my adrenaline skyrocketing with the excitement of the moment. I scanned the crowd until I spotted my husband, Jack, and 17-year-old daughter, Lindsey, giving me huge smiles and shouts of encouragement.

The crowd was screaming and cheering. My heart was beating like it wanted to jump out of my chest, as torch number 141 was handed to me. Security police on motorcycles flanked each of the torchbearers.

Each of the officers had keys on black lanyards around their necks to unlock the propane vent on the torches. The security policeman to my left opened the propane canister with his key, placed his hands on my shoulders, guiding me to the center of the street, facing backward toward the relay runner.

We had been instructed to lean our torches toward the upcoming runner. As he approached me, we angled our torches, similar to toasting a glass of wine. The flame jumped from his torch to light mine. One of the officers quickly extinguished torch 140 by turning off the propane with the same key used to start up mine, then blew out the remaining flame. This all happened in a matter of seconds.

I turned around as the crowd shouted, "Go, Tamy!"

Starting up the 15-grade hill, feeling almost breathless, I heard my friends yell, "Slow down, Tamy. You're not a runner, you're a walker, and besides, we want to get pictures." I quickly obeyed.

The torch was heavier than I expected. I didn't want to drop it. We had chanted as a group on the shuttle bus, "Don't drop the torch!" I needed to carry it almost straight-armed in front of me. The wind was so strong that the flame was blowing flat and looked as if it might catch my hat on fire.

I ran/walked a total of three-tenths of a mile, knowing that I wasn't running just for myself but for all of the women who were fighting breast cancer. I was running for my wonderful family and friends, for all cancer survivors, and for friends and family I had lost to this horrid disease.

That was also true in April when I received the Spirit of Survivorship Carpe Diem Award from the Lance Armstrong Foundation. Once again, my family and closest friends (whom I call my guardian angels) flew down to Austin, Texas, in support as I accepted this award from Lance.

While I feel honored to have had the opportunity to carry the Olympic torch and to receive the Survivorship Award, I believe there is a higher purpose for my continuing to survive with stage 4 breast cancer. To have the ability to encourage others to remain positive and live life to its fullest despite their prognosis, I believe, is my God-given purpose now. As one of the longest surviving bone marrow transplant recipients (30 years) and for living with stage 4 breast cancer for over six years, I think God has plans for me to continue in service to others.

To HAVE THE ABILITY to encourage others to remain positive and live life to its fullest despite their prognosis, I believe, is my God-given purpose now.

My personal motto is "Celebrate life every day."

I have had a wonderful life so far, and it just keeps getting better.

Look Good, Feel Better

Because I've been a cosmetologist for 41 years, I have plenty of customers and my appointment book is always packed. But I have to say that one of my favorite appointments is the second Wednesday of every month. That's when I offer free services to other breast cancer survivors like myself, many of whom recently have lost or are about to lose their hair as a result of chemotherapy treatments.

I know firsthand what it's like trying to figure out how to cover a bald head, how to fabricate eyebrows that are no longer there, and how to use foundation to correct blotchy skin from chemotherapy and radiation.

At the beginning of a free two-hour makeup and skin care session at the Sacramento American Cancer Society office, I greet the women who have arrived at what I like to think of as a pajama party without the sleepover. "Come on in," I urge them. "Find a place at the conference table, and I'll explain how to use all of the cosmetics in the makeup kits before you."

As the women of all ages and ethnicities take their places at the table, I can hear them connecting by talking about their cancer experiences. Each place setting has a placemat, a pink standup mirror with two sides including a magnifier, and a kit filled with makeup and skin care products. Once everyone is seated, I begin the program. "Hello, everyone. My name is Bev Nason, and eight years ago I could have been in a session just like this because I am a breast cancer survivor."

I can see smiles forming on their faces because they know that one of their own is leading the group.

From experience, I am aware that there are three different groups of women in the room. Some are newly diagnosed and don't know what will happen and they've come to seek knowledge. I see another group, women wearing wigs, and a third group are those who are done with the chemotherapy and radiation and don't want to go back to work without eyebrows.

I SEE HOW HAPPY the women are with their new looks. Their faces reveal that there are beautiful souls on the inside.

After the women take off their old makeup, a 12-step makeup application begins. I use a volunteer model to show them how to make eyebrows almost magically appear thanks to the help of connecting dots strategically placed with an eyebrow pencil. "Your eyes are a window to your soul," I tell them as they look into their mirrors and add color to their eyelids.

I've been volunteering for this program for the past five years, and I have felt so fulfilled, probably more than the "students" have, because I have given them the techniques to regain their attractive appearance. At the end of the class, I see how happy the women are with their new looks. Their faces reveal that there are beautiful souls on the inside, and they truly are a reflection of the program's name: Look Good, Feel Better.

We all do.

Susan King

I Have Become a Dragon Slayer

With stage 3 breast cancer at the age of 45, I decided to start each day by looking in the mirror, making eye contact, and saying to myself out loud, "Yes, you may die, but not today."

That was the way I was able to keep focused on the present and not venture into the unknown and scary future.

Treatment began quickly after my diagnosis, which had transformed me from a supermom to a sick, tired, and emotional mother of three children. (I wanted to start treatment as soon as possible to be rid of the dragon growing and multiplying inside of me.)

I had four rounds of chemotherapy before the surgery to remove my right breast. After the surgery, the doctors suggested four more rounds of chemotherapy and a stem cell transplant.

Having a stem cell transplant was the hardest decision I ever had to make. It came with great risks and was a terrible assault of poisons in my body. I prayed to God to give me a sign about whether it would be a good idea to go ahead with the controversial treatment. My only sign, I realized, was there were no roadblocks in my way. "You have to do this," I told myself, "because you won't ever want to look back and wish you had."

When I checked into the hospital for a month-long stay, I had all of my important things around me, like pictures of my family, my children's drawings, a religious medal, a friendship heart, and a lion for courage my aunt had given me.

As the chemotherapy began through a port in my chest, I envisioned myself as a warrior, a single-breasted woman with a shield of will. I would take my poison with dignity. I would not let the dragon destroy my hope, my will, and my life.

Although I was wretched with illness from the medicine, I would imagine myself strong, my hand firmly grasping my staff, which I held high. A silver cross was my poison as I ex-orcised the dragon from my body. Defeat would not over-take me. I had come far to meet this enemy before me.

I HAVE BECOME THE dragon slayer and my cells are cancer-free. I have fought this war and won.

When I looked at myself in the mirror, I saw a woman standing proud, even though I had no hair and was naked and cold. I said to the dragon and myself with conviction, "I will live to be an old woman. I will never have cancer again."

I have become the dragon slayer and my cells are cancer-free. I have fought this war and won.

I have learned that life is never more important until it is being taken from you. I have written down all of my dreams, and I have strived to make them come true, like seeing the

Grand Canyon, writing children's books, teaching mosaic art classes, and taking creative writing courses.

I would never have reached this point if it weren't for the Wellness Community, a place where people meet in small groups with a counselor to share their experiences with the disease of cancer. I learned to talk openly about fear and about death as we comforted each other, including those who were dying. Another source of strength was the love and prayers from my family and friends.

One day when I looked at the sky after a fresh-smelling rain, I saw a rainbow God had painted and I knew that he was promising me another tomorrow—and I was thankful.

The Music of My Life

L isten," I told my surgeon right before my mastectomy. "Before the anesthesia is administered, I would
like you to play a cassette of music and positive affirmations I've made for myself. I want to hear the tape as I
go under."

The music with a strong beat filled the operating room,
beckoning the warrior within me to stand ready for the battle
against cancer. Intermixed were affirmations in my voice like,
"My body is strengthened and renewed" and "A part of me is
gone but I am more whole now than ever."

I heard the tape when I was sedated by the anesthesia and
when I awoke from the surgery.

If you knew me, you'd know that the tape request wasn't
unusual. Music has played an enormous part in my life, like
the time I moved to New York City and operated an off, off-
Broadway theater company. Not knowing anyone in the city
except for the people with whom I worked, I turned to music
for companionship, whether it was in my lower, trash-can

level, studio apartment in Manhattan or when I was walking the busy streets in the city.

The year was 1997, and I was a strong, successful, independent woman living in Sacramento who had proved that I could take care of myself. It doesn't work that way with cancer, though. All of my life, I could do anything I set my mind to, but with cancer, I couldn't make it go away or call on the folks or a friend to do the job for me.

After spending three days immediately following diagnosis in a cocoon of terror inside my home, I dealt with hatred, anger, and just about every negative emotion in the spectrum. I came to a realization that I can be present in this experience by creating a positive living environment and I can feel joyful for another day to live.

Music became a source of comfort and a call to action when I spent many hours at home. The music I listened, sang, or hummed to changed depending on my mood. Sometimes it was a John Philip Sousa march that would help me get in touch with my strength and courage to fight this disease. Other times, Medwyn Goodall would help me with the sounds of *Medicine Woman*, soothing music from flutes and tribal rhythms celebrating the power of nurturing and healing. Or, in times of strength and courage, Nicholas Gunn's *Sacred Fire* empowered me with percussion beats and stirring vocals burning with the intensity of primitive dance.

Dance movement therapy helped me get in touch with my spirit.

Dance movement therapy helped me get in touch with my spirit. "What do you want to get out of this class?" Nandi, the class leader, asked.

"I just want to feel okay with this body and hear the music," I told her.

In a big, drab, pink and mottled gray conference room at a cancer center in Sacramento, 10 women, all of us strangers, all of us cancer survivors, gathered around Nandi and her boom box. "Welcome, beauties," I heard Nandi say.

I thought, "Oh, my God. I don't know if I can stand this," and at the same time, "Oh, my God, we are all beauties; we are women survivors of cancer."

Nandi told us that if the music speaks to us and if we want to move to it, we should go right ahead. She also said, "Love yourself, your whole self, the part of your body that has been affected by cancer."

At first, I just watched people slowly moving, their bodies swaying. Within a few minutes, I found myself moving, too, unconsciously breathing rhythmically to the beat of the music. The session lasted two hours and I didn't want it to end because the combination of the music and the movement helped me realize that I could and would be okay even though a part of this woman's body, my breast, was gone.

I attended those classes each Tuesday and Thursday for 12 weeks, and when they were over, their lessons stayed with me, helping me recognize the completeness of my new being and embrace the spirit and power of today and the vision and dreams of tomorrow.

Five years after my recovery, a group of us from Nandi's class performed at a reunion. With a sense of victory, pride, and exuberance, we moved our beautiful and whole bodies to the song "Stayin' Alive" from the movie *Saturday Night Fever:* "Ooh, ooh, ooh, ooh, stayin' alive, stayin' alive."

That said it all.

Jeannie Paslawsky

Turning a Whisper into a Roar

Once upon a time, there was a beautiful woman. She was a kind and lovely lady. One day, a frightening Beast came along and stole her away. It kept her prisoner and fought off all attempts to rescue her.

Day after day, every three minutes, a fine woman, loved by many, is diagnosed with breast cancer. Each woman is captured by a Beast that steals her away for months at a time, sometimes forever. Each one of these women is deeply loved; she is someone's daughter, mom, sister, wife, grandmother, aunt, and girlfriend.

* * *

In January 1999, I called my dear friend Jean Walsh, who told me, "Oh, Jeannie, I have breast cancer." I barely heard the next several hours of conversation, my head still reeling from her first news. Immediately I wanted to know what I could do. Not much, I have learned, sharing Jean's personal journey every day since then. Despite the distance, we stay in touch like neighbors. We e-mail daily and call often to "visit," and I have written "real mail" cards and letters to her, sometimes daily if she were particularly sick or down. When she told me how much the mail helped her, I always answered: "Sure they do, Jean, *real mail* is good medicine."

Over time, in my feeble attempts to walk on this journey with Jean, I have read her online support boards and come to know and love many of the modern lovely ladies fighting the Beast. Unlike the Fairy Tales, where rescuers are heroes, these ladies are *my* heroes. After treatments, they go to PTO meetings and to their kids' baseball and soccer games, not caring that they are sick. They attend weddings and graduations without hair, gratefully rejoicing to be there. They make lunches despite the nausea. They even joke about things like the number of stitches from surgery. They celebrate every holiday and birthday with a bittersweet tear known quietly to them. And they somehow smile through it all.

Each one of these women is deeply loved; she is someone's daughter, mom, sister, wife, grandmother, aunt, and girlfriend.

By April 2000, the Beast had spread to Jean's bones, metastasized; again I had *to do something*. In September 2000, her local "BC (breast cancer) mentor" had died. That was something no one had expected. Jean called me in October: "Jeannie, I am *sick* of this disease. We need to stop whispering about breast cancer! We need to ROAR!"

October, which is National Breast Cancer Awareness Month, is very hard for these heroes of mine. Jean and her online "BC Sisters" talked online about their hurt and disappointment over the usual October messages. "Catch it early" they were told. They were also enraged because the breast cancer stories covered "NED" (No Evidence of Disease) survivors, not those surviving as they were, battling the beast daily or weekly with chemo, trying to stave it off, to prevent progression further past the bones (or eyes, or lungs, or liver), pushing back the inevitable as long as they could. Sometimes, *too many times,* once every 12 minutes, the Beast wins.

All this time, *everyday*, I wanted to *do something*. It was early that October when Jean asked me if I could help her. Her idea was to collect 1 million letters asking the president for more federal funding for breast cancer research. Since then, we have been "ROARing for a Cure." We received more than 11,000 letters in our first six weeks, letters written by those with breast cancer and those who share their fight.

The ROAR has now evolved into many forms: original letters written in schools and homes and the thousands of preprinted letters and petitions signed at work, cancer runs and walks, parties, and community gatherings. In April 2002, the ROAR Campaign joined another endeavor to raise breast cancer awareness: a cross-country bicycle ride from California to Florida, "Cycling for a Cure." Our ROAR got louder as I worked PR for the four women cyclists of Terre Haute, Indiana. Led by Lori Ugo, they rode daily, climbing mountains and crossing deserts to spread the word about breast cancer and the need for research funds for a cure. They traveled along Route I-10 from San Diego, California, to St. Augustine, Florida. Each night Lori updated me and I sent a press release to newspaper, radio, and television editors. The cyclists, like me, are not survivors but are *doing something* anyway.

Awareness is not publicity. Raising awareness for breast cancer is asking someone to sign a letter for breast cancer research funding and that person then saying, "Yes, because I know . . ." (going on to name a name), or a teary, "Oh, sure. Mom died of breast cancer. Can I help?" Awareness is asking folks at an October football game to stand if they never knew anyone with breast cancer; then looking around to see that everyone remained seated. It is ROARing from a rooftop. It is the U-go riders (named after organizer Lori Ugo) distributing breast cancer literature and ROAR Campaign letters at every campground, truck stop, and small town grocery store or diner along the way—Turning the Whisper into a ROAR.

Over time, we've met many others who, like me, have wanted to *do something* to fight the breast cancer Beast. We are *not* in a fairy tale and this Beast is very strong; too often there is no "happy ending." Our voices must overpower it . . . we must do something to find a cure—*for my heroes!*

* * *

Do something! Come visit http://www.arborontheweb .com/roar/ for more information.

Sandy Smoley

Going Public with Breast Cancer

hen I was first diagnosed with breast cancer, I didn't believe it and neither did my doctor. The diagnosis came as a result of testing my breast tissue after a surgery. Prior to the surgery, I had a mammogram and all the testing turned up clear; so when the breast tissue came back as positive for cancer, both my doctor and I were in shock.

This was the mid-1980s. At the time, I was beginning my third of what was to be five four-year terms as county supervisor. My career as a public figure was growing, and serving my community became increasingly important to me.

I was the very first woman in Sacramento to be elected to a county office. I thought at the time that having breast cancer while holding a public office would be about the worst thing that could happen.

The doctor had the tissue sent to specialists at Sloan Kettering Cancer Hospital. The results were positive. Now the agonizing decision about how to handle my illness was looming before me.

At that time, breast cancer was not talked about openly. Never before had an elected official dealt with breast cancer publicly. Of course, in the 1980s, there weren't too many women in publicly held offices either. Any choice I made was a risk to my community service.

My initial reaction was to be very, very quiet about the entire ordeal. It was difficult enough for me to accept this new realization; I could not imagine how the public would feel. Nor did I particularly want to face the potential feelings of disrespect in a predominantly male world. In the end, what changed my mind was the strength I knew I would gain by going public with my illness.

It was 14 days after the positive diagnosis that I was scheduled for a double mastectomy. By telling women all over the county what I was about to face, I discovered a sense of courage that gave me incredible strength. The *Sacramento Bee* ran my story as one of the feature articles on their cover; radio stations and television stations all over the county covered the news.

On the actual day of my surgery, local television reporters set up outside the hospital to report on my progress. Once the surgery was complete, a press conference was held with my husband, my doctor, and one of my closest friends. The message that I was diagnosed, and then endured the agony of the operation publicly, became an inspiration for women all across northern California. Many of them approached me in public and told me so.

Today, 17 years later, I still recall how difficult that decision was for me. To go public in a time when breast cancer just wasn't talked about openly was the right decision. So many women have made a point to personally tell me that my ordeal motivated them to seek a mammogram or even ask for more testing in a situation that was unclear. To this day I continue to speak at breast cancer forums and fundraising events. My message is clear and simple: Be assertive and take charge of your health.

Get mammograms, do breast self-exams, and do whatever you have to do to face your future with courage. If you are not satisfied with your doctor's diagnosis, get another doctor

> *If you are not satisfied with your doctor's diagnosis, get another doctor or absolutely insist on further testing.*

or absolutely insist on further testing. Each of us has a well of strength that we can tap into; find yours and use it, regardless of what anyone might think.

When my ordeal was over and I was finally deemed "cured," I drove through the streets of downtown Sacramento, radio at full blast, the window down on my car, and I screamed at the top of my lungs, "I'm cured! I'm cured!"

Judy Lewis

Early Detection Was My Goal

My mother and my aunt had breast cancer. So there was little doubt in my mind that one day I, too, could be diagnosed with breast cancer. Of course I didn't want to get cancer, so I was determined to watch for any early warning signals. Being vigilant gave me strength. I became a sentry with the mission of being on the lookout for an approaching enemy. I didn't want to be the victim of a surprise attack.

I had lumpy breasts to begin with, so in addition to getting an annual mammogram, my gynecologist recommended that I see a surgeon to check my breasts on a regular basis. During those visits, the surgeon used a syringe with an inch-long needle to drain the lumps. No matter how many lumps he drained, they always returned within a month.

The procedure was uncomfortable, both physically and emotionally. I cringed every time I received an appointment reminder postcard, and for days before the appointment, I anguished over going to the surgeon's office. But I always returned. In my heart and head I knew that I couldn't win the battle if I didn't do everything medically possible to conquer cancer before it had a chance to overtake me.

One visit, as I lay on the tissue-covered examining table for the umpteenth time, the surgeon found a lump in my left breast that he didn't like. He sent me for a mammogram. That dreadful visit proved more valuable than ever. I felt like I had spent years waiting in line on a relay team for someone to finally pass me the baton. Now it had been handed to me and it was my turn to run with it.

Because early detection had always been my goal, I felt well equipped to face the battle. I felt confident that my diligence would pay off and it did. A biopsy showed a small 0.7-centimeter tumor. It was now time to deal with the reality of a mastectomy and whatever subsequent treatment was warranted.

Yes, breast cancer is scary, but even while I was going through the process, I felt like a success story.

Although the cancer was found in only one breast, I decided to have a double mastectomy and reconstruction. I've never regretted that decision; in addition to the targeted tumor, the pathology showed additional cancer cells within the same breast. Furthermore, I had figured it would be just a matter of time before cancer would develop in the second breast, and I didn't want to have to go through this again. I was rewarded for my diligence. The removal of my lymph nodes showed that the cancer hadn't spread. This fact, combined with the small size of the tumor, allowed me to avoid radiation and chemotherapy.

From diagnosis to surgery to recovery, I maintained a positive attitude. While my supportive circle of family, friends, and doctors was profoundly important, so was the knowledge that I was approaching this with the deck stacked in my favor. Knowing that I did everything I could to detect the cancer early eased my mind and gave me strength to get through the mastectomies. Yes, breast cancer is scary, but even while I was going through the process, I felt like a success story.

It has been almost two years since the diagnosis of my breast cancer. The recovery from my surgery went so quickly that I was back at work, part-time, after just two weeks. I'm 50 years old and I'm living proof that the best defense is a good offense.

Online Support

I look in the mirror and smirk at my reflection. I have HAIR! So what if I look like Curly Sue? Just a few months ago, I looked like GI Jane. I was glad to see *that* look go out of style! But this mop? "Chemo curls," that's what I call them.

I go to the computer and sign on to www.delphi.com/made it/messages—a forum. I head straight to 'Breast Cancer Survivors and Friends' where I have my own cyberspace support group. I wonder what's happening today.

* * *

Eighteen months ago, I found the Breast Cancer Survivors and Friends forum while searching online for something that I desperately needed to know—"What was the prognosis for a 36-year-old woman with breast cancer?" I typed 'breast cancer' into the rectangular search box on my computer screen and scanned the list of possible Web sites. I found a list of breast cancer incidents by location. Ohio was a hot spot of cancers. Not reassuring. I kept searching, trying different variations; 'chemotherapy,' 'survival,' 'prognosis,' on and on.

Then, I found myself on WebMD.com, viewing the message boards. I clicked on one and read about a woman interested in tamoxifen information. Another woman was wondering if her side effects were normal. Then, I read a message from a woman named Brandie, asking anyone with breast cancer or a friend with breast cancer to come to her forum. She was recently diagnosed with breast cancer herself. Out of curiosity, I went to her forum. There I found messages and comments from women just like me. The women visiting the site were of varying ages, locations, and backgrounds, and the treatments were as varied as we were. Some had had lumpectomies, some mastectomies; some chemo, and others radiation or a combination of both.

Brandie wrote that she had not started chemotherapy, but knew what kind she would be getting. Others who had the same chemotherapy drugs reassured her by telling her about their experiences, including side effects and recovery.

I didn't find the answer I was looking for then, and maybe I never will. But what I have found is a group of women who share the same disease that I do. We share the same emotional turmoil, body changes, medication hassles, physician and oncologist visits. We share the same fears. We share our happiness and our joys. When I ask, "Know what I mean?" I know they do.

I don't feel so alone anymore!

It has been three and a half years since I was diagnosed with breast cancer. I underwent a mastectomy and reconstruction. I endured the loss of my hair and the forced menopause. I have been through every emotion that a woman can imagine with this disease. And, I have survived!

What matters to me now is acceptance of my situation and a desire to help other women under 40 who have been diagnosed with breast cancer. Big things can be accomplished by sharing what we have been through and telling others how we can cope. Forums are a great way to offer support and caring thoughts as we share what we know and feel with our friends in cyberspace and in person.

I wrote this poem to reflect my feelings about online support groups:

Big things can be accomplished by sharing what we have been through and telling others how we can cope.

Search Engines
Search the universe for
*   the answer to this*
I contemplate the seriousness of my situation
To those who have been there
And to those who return
I ask you, share your wisdom, share your knowledge
My fear grows from the unknown
With the answers hidden from me
I am bombarded with irrelevant information
But what I need are hard facts
Before I go insane
From the lack of unorganized searching
My own resources fail me severely
And I weep the tears of the frustrated
Who only needs this one answer
Who only needs a good, solid hug
To gather myself up and continue my search
for it's all I have now.

Never Be Defeated

It had been 18 years since the leukemia, the chemotherapy, and the bone marrow transplant. Life had been hard at times, but I was feeling good at the age of 38 and optimistic about the future. I was married to a good man, and we were excited about his recent job promotion. After years of waiting, our dreams of buying a house and adopting a baby felt within reach.

One day, while doing my routine monthly breast exam, I felt a lump. I was puzzled but not frightened. I was feeling too healthy to have anything seriously wrong, and I had finally let go of the fear of recurring cancer. "Surely, it's nothing important," I reassured myself. But to be on the responsible and safe side, I had a mammogram. No one could have been more surprised than I was that the lump turned out to be a three-centimeter tumor.

The bad news made me angry, disappointed, and overwhelmed, all at the same time. What about all of our dreams? Peter and I had known that I couldn't get pregnant after the bone marrow transplant and we accepted that, knowing that we could easily love an adopted baby. Now our dreams were shattered, and I was afraid of what the future would hold.

The fear I felt was not new to me because I remembered all too well what it took to fight the leukemia, and the thought of a mastectomy, of possibly needing chemotherapy, and the fear of the cancer spreading were horrifying. I wondered if I could face cancer all over again. Could I fight this battle and win? What were the odds of winning twice?

The upcoming breast surgery seemed so barbaric, and my heart would leap in panic when I thought of the cancer growing like an invading enemy inside my body. The only way I could calm down was to take long walks that summer in my Seattle neighborhood and to talk to God, thanking him for all that was wonderful in my world. "Thank you, for life, for 18 years more than any doctor had promised me and for Peter who loves me just the way I am. You have helped me through so much, and now I need your help again. Please keep the cancer from spreading so I can get well, and help me to fight this disease with dignity."

God did not give me the leukemia or the breast cancer. People get sick; that is just a fact of life. Life is not fair. It never was and it never will be. I had learned many things from the last illness, and I could learn from this, too. Yes, I would have to change my plans again, but I was trusting God to have another plan in mind. Somehow in my life, I would find a way to be happy and to make a difference.

Religious music played a role in my healing. When I went to the health club to walk on the treadmill, I would put on my headphones and turn up the music. One of my favorite songs was by Dion, called "Hymn to Him" on the album *Velvet and Steel*.

. . . If the winds of disaster have blown hard through your night and

the dreams you have cherished can't begin to take flight.

Take His hand through the sunlight.

Lift your head high above.

Let your heart flow forever with the warmth of His love . . .

As I listened to the music, I placed one foot after the other. With each step I felt more determined, and I could feel my shoulders relax and my chin come up. I was ready to fight this disease again and again, if need be. The sadness that I seemed to carry around with me lifted—I was ready for the challenge. I was going to meet this new cancer head-on and see who would win this round.

> ⟡ THE SADNESS THAT *I seemed to carry around with me lifted—I was ready for the challenge. I was going to meet this new cancer head-on and see who would win this round.*

Uncertain of the direction I should take for my recovery, I got more than one opinion on my options. I chose an oncologist who had a good reputation, who did thorough exams, who took time to answer my questions, and who I felt comfortable with. I followed his advice and had a modified radical mastectomy.

The lab reports came back and they were not good. The cancer was aggressive, estrogen positive, and had spread to one lymph node out of 22. When I was advised to do chemotherapy, the dread and anger surfaced all over again. I had struggled so many years from the heavy dosages of chemo for the leukemia and the three hours of total body radiation for the transplant, that I just could not see myself doing chemotherapy again. Even though my oncologist assured me that the chemo for breast cancer was much lower than what I had for the bone marrow transplant, I just couldn't do it. I was taking a dangerously high risk that the cancer had not gotten further than one lymph node, but at that time in my life, that was a risk I was willing to take. I did concede, however, to taking tamoxifen, and I set out to become as healthy as I could be on my own.

A friend of mine recommended a counselor whom she liked and with whom I found a safe place to let go of my anger and fear. Each week I would arrive feeling weighed down and leave feeling drained of bad feelings and much more relaxed, like I had just been swimming—a good kind of tired and very clean.

A friend told me about a naturopath who practiced Nogier Auricular Medicine. It is an energetic diagnostic and treatment technique that reveals the cause of illness and allows the practitioner to diagnose on a cause level, not just a symptoms level. Using homeopathic remedies specifically for my needs, she was able to detoxify my body and build up my immune system.

I studied and followed an anticancer diet, and I stayed away from foods to which I was either allergic or sensitive. I stopped eating the small amount of sugar and chocolate I enjoyed and was thankful that I never liked coffee or wine. I went ahead and spent the extra money for organic foods and purified water.

I was introduced to a Qi Gong master, who worked with me for a year without charge just because he was so worried about me. I practiced Qi Gong, which is a Chinese form of gentle movement, to regain health and to balance my energy, or Qi. I found the best time for me to do my Qi Gong was in the morning out in my backyard. In the winter, I would wear gloves, a scarf, and a hat and bundle up with layers of clothes, my black sweatpants on the bottom and my bulky, royal blue jacket on top. After a while, even the rain upon my face felt wonderful. At times I would close my eyes and hear all the sounds around me. I would focus on how my body was feeling as I ever so slowly would raise my arms to the sky and then slowly lower them in different patterns, breathing all the while into my abdomen. On clear days, when the sun shone upon my face, I would think of it as God's life-giving energy shining down on me, giving me energy and healing.

I went on long, happy walks with one of my girlfriends through all kinds of weather, and I met a new friend who was also fighting cancer. I did not feel so alone and overwhelmed when we teamed up to share support and information on procedures, doctors, anticancer diets, and recipes.

I had such a need to record all that I was feeling and learning that I started taking time to keep a journal. Having this quiet time to reflect, grow, and feel connected to God helped me to recover. In my journal I wrote about fear, faith, and forgiveness. For example, on December 2, 1996, five months into my recovery, I wrote, "Fear can be such a debilitating thing. It can take the time I have left to live and steal even that away if I let it. . . . Life is like a classroom. Some have harder classes for a while but it seems to all even out in the end." I've reached the conclusion that cancer is just one of the many tragedies in this world that somehow seems to give clarity to one's mind. The unimportant details in my life took the back seat for a while, and the simple things—like feeling well, laughing, being with those I love, and forgiving past wrongs—were seen in a whole new light.

I learned that when I slowed down, time seemed to slow down. I found that I could either learn to swim or drown in the storms life sends my way. I also realized that I could learn and grow from disappointment and adversity if I chose to. I decided that if the cancer took over, if I died from this, I would not have failed. I would only fail if I lost my faith in God, if I didn't see what was truly important in life, and if I didn't forgive others for past wrongs or myself for mistakes I had made. I decided that for as long as I could, I would square my shoulders and continue forward, being kind, giving, and courageous.

As I write this, I have been cancer-free for six and a half years. Peter and I have enjoyed living in our own little house with our animal kids. Peter runs a hotel and I am pursuing a career in art. We will not be adopting because my energy level is still too low, but we will be enjoying our nieces and nephews.

Even though I am cancer-free, I have not lost the value of its lessons. I still look around and see things in a new way. I love to listen to great music because it lifts my mood. Some-

I DECIDED THAT for as long as I could, I would square my shoulders and continue forward, being kind, giving, and courageous.

times I sing songs in my car as I drive, and I don't mind if others see me looking a bit foolish, singing out loud and tapping the steering wheel.

Each day, I try to remember to live life fully and to see life as a journey. I treasure my family, friends, and pets. I laugh at good jokes and hold on to my faith. Sometimes, when the day is done, I turn and face the horizon, deeply breathing in the evening air. I watch the sun slide out of sight as I hold my head up high, thanking God for allowing me to live another day. I hold on to this time, hold on to my faith in God, and know in my heart and soul that whether in life or death, I will never be defeated.